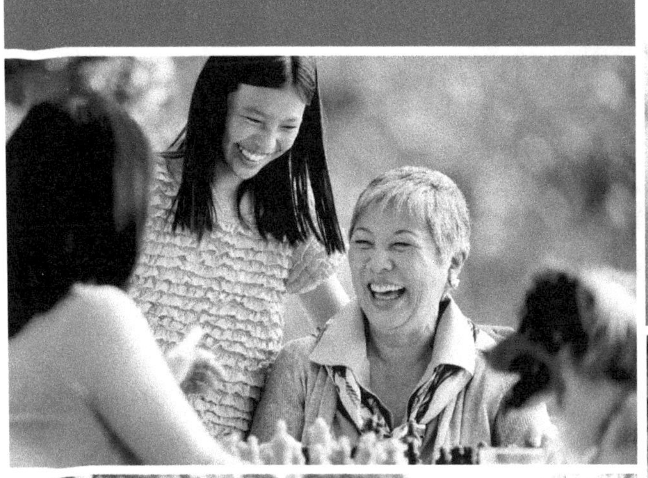

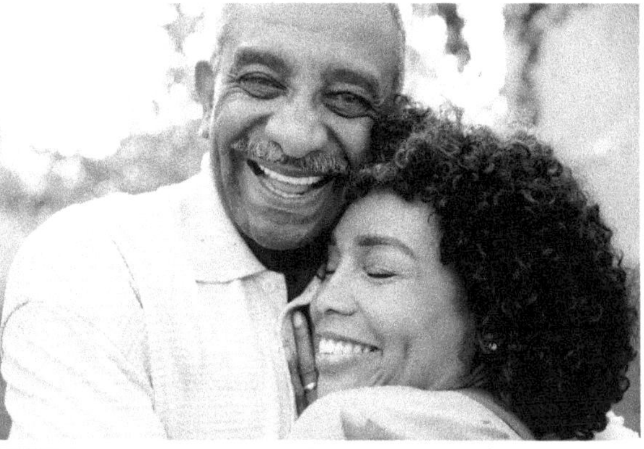

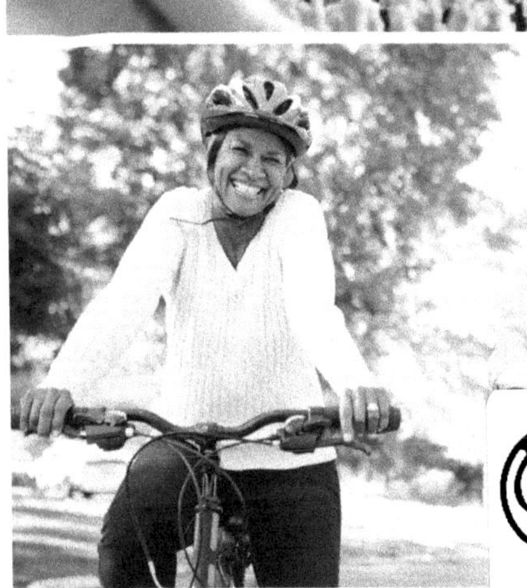

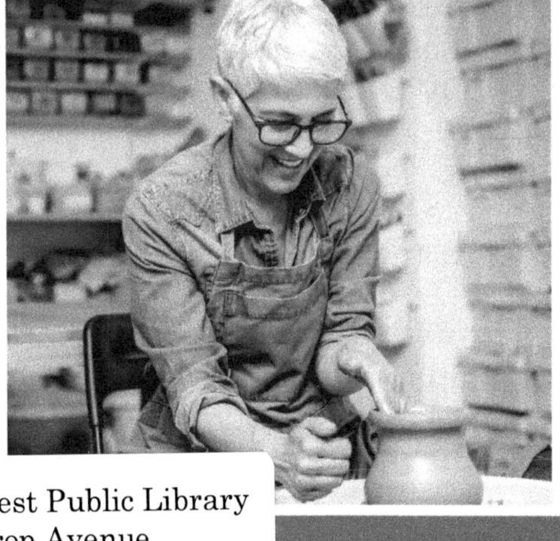

Medicare & You 2023

The official U.S. government Medicare handbook

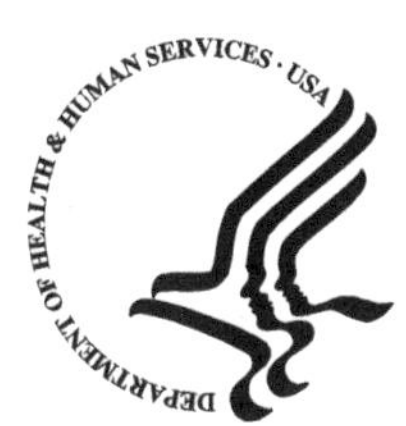

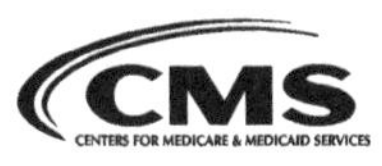

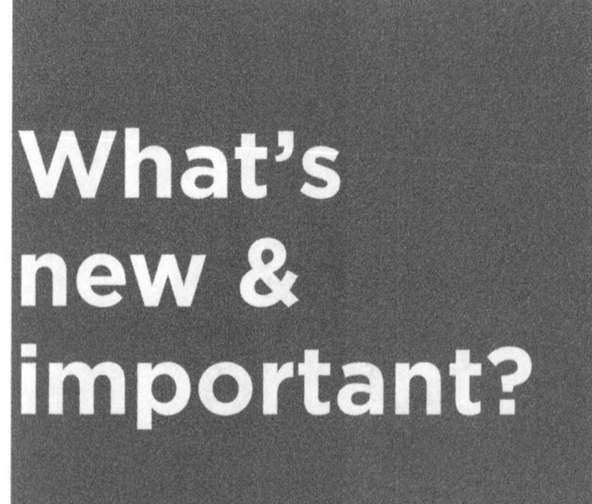

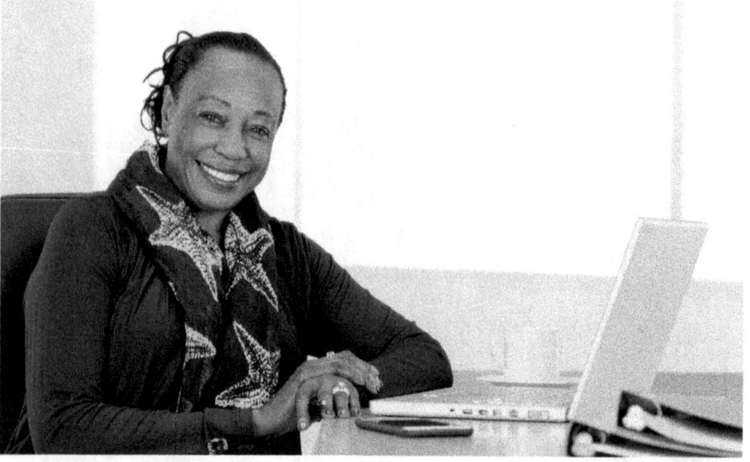

COVID-19 updates
Medicare continues to cover several tests, items, and services related to the coronavirus disease 2019 (COVID-19). See pages 37–38.

Another time to sign up for Medicare
You might be able to sign up for Medicare during a Special Enrollment Period if you missed your enrollment period because of certain exceptional circumstances. See page 18.

New start dates for your Medicare coverage
When you sign up for Medicare the month you turn 65 or during the last 3 months of your Initial Enrollment Period, or during the General Enrollment Period, your coverage starts the first day of the month after you sign up. See pages 17–18.

Kidney transplants & immunosuppressive drug coverage
Medicare offers a benefit that helps you pay for your immunosuppressive drugs beyond 36 months after a kidney transplant (if you don't have certain types of other health coverage). See page 53.

Learn how Accountable Care Organizations are driving better health care
An Accountable Care Organization is a group of doctors, hospitals, and other health care providers that have teamed up to give you coordinated health care. If your doctor is part of an Accountable Care Organization, it means you may have access to additional benefits focused on your needs. See pages 111–112.

Get help paying your Medicare health and drug costs
If you have limited income, you may be able to get help from your state to pay your Medicare costs through resources like Extra Help or a Medicare Savings Program. See pages 91–96.

Get help in a crisis
Your mental health and wellness are a high priority. If you or someone you know is in crisis, call or text 988, or chat 988lifeline.org.

Need information in an accessible format or another language?
You can get the "Medicare & You" handbook in an accessible format at no cost to you. See page 123. To get free help in a language other than English, see pages 125-126.

Contents

Looking for the Index of topics?
See page 4.

Symbol key
Look for these symbols throughout this handbook to help you understand your Medicare coverage:

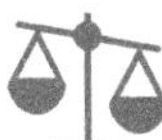
Compare: Shows comparisons between Original Medicare and Medicare Advantage Plans.

Cost & coverage: Gives you information about costs and coverage for services.

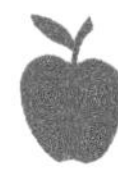
Preventive service: Gives you details about preventive services.

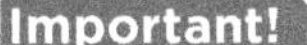

Important: Highlights information that's important to review.

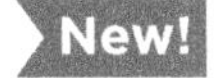

New: Highlights what's new in this year's "Medicare & You."

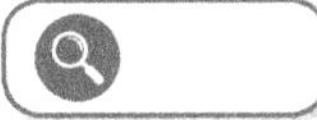
Helps you find important information on Medicare.gov.

Index of topics

A

B

C

Note: The **bold** page numbers have the most details.

D

E

F

G

H

Note: The **bold** page numbers have the most details.

Note: The **bold** page numbers have the most details.

N

O

P

Q

R

Note: The **bold** page numbers have the most details.

S

T

U

V

W

X

Note: The **bold** page numbers have the most details.

What are the parts of Medicare?

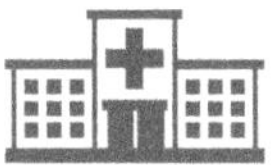

Part A (Hospital Insurance)

Helps cover:

- Inpatient care in hospitals
- Skilled nursing facility care
- Hospice care
- Home health care

See pages 25–29.

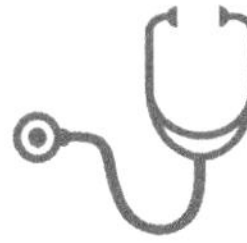

Part B (Medical Insurance)

Helps cover:

- Services from doctors and other health care providers
- Outpatient care
- Home health care
- Durable medical equipment (like wheelchairs, walkers, hospital beds, and other equipment)
- Many preventive services (like screenings, shots or vaccines, and yearly "Wellness" visits)

See pages 29–55.

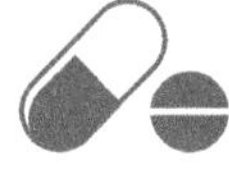

Part D (Drug coverage)

Helps cover the cost of prescription drugs (including many recommended shots or vaccines).

Plans that offer Medicare drug coverage (Part D) are run by private insurance companies that follow rules set by Medicare.

See pages 79–90.

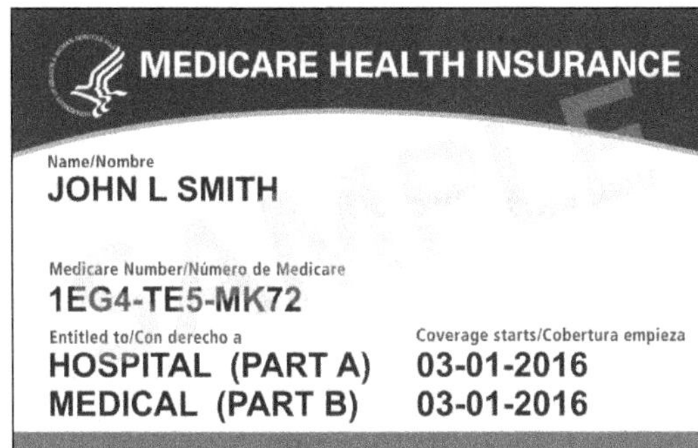

Replace your Medicare card

Need to replace a damaged or lost Medicare card? Log into (or create) your secure Medicare account at Medicare.gov to print or order an official copy of your Medicare card. You can also call 1-800-MEDICARE (1-800-633-4227) and ask for a replacement card to be sent in the mail. TTY users can call 1-877-486-2048.

If you get Railroad Retirement Board (RRB) benefits, you can call 1-877-772-5772 to get a replacement card. TTY users can call 1-312-751-4701.

Your Medicare options

When you first sign up for Medicare, and during certain times of the year, you can choose how you get your Medicare coverage. There are 2 main ways to get Medicare:

Original Medicare

- Original Medicare includes Medicare Part A (Hospital Insurance) and Part B (Medical Insurance).
- You can join a separate Medicare drug plan to get Medicare drug coverage (Part D).
- You can use any doctor or hospital that takes Medicare, anywhere in the U.S.
- To help pay your out-of-pocket costs in Original Medicare (like your 20% coinsurance), you can also shop for and buy supplemental coverage.

☑ **Part A**

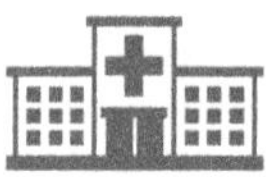

☑ **Part B**

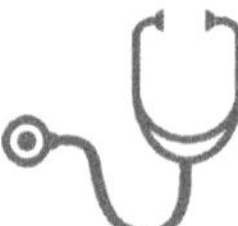

You can add:

☐ **Part D**

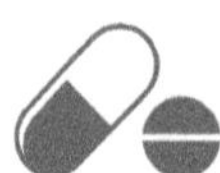

You can also add:

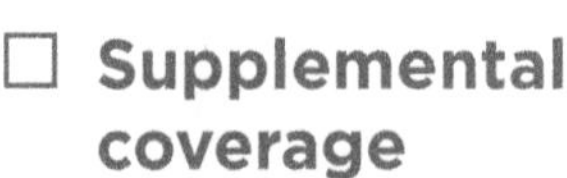

☐ **Supplemental coverage**

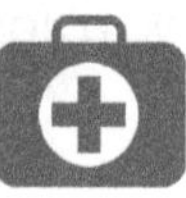

This includes Medicare Supplement Insurance (Medigap). See Section 5 (starting on page 75) to learn more about Medigap. Or, you can use coverage from a former employer or union, or Medicaid.

See Section 3 (starting on page 57) to learn more about Original Medicare.

Medicare Advantage

(also known as Part C)

- Medicare Advantage is a Medicare-approved plan from a private company that offers an alternative to Original Medicare for your health and drug coverage. These "bundled" plans include Part A, Part B, and usually Part D.
- In most cases, you can only use doctors who are in the plan's network.
- In many cases, you may need to get approval from your plan before it covers certain drugs or services.
- Plans may have lower out-of-pocket costs than Original Medicare.
- Plans may offer some extra benefits that Original Medicare doesn't cover—like vision, hearing, and dental services.

☑ **Part A**

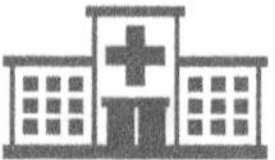

☑ **Part B**

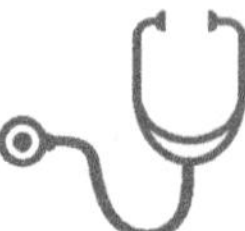

Most plans include:

☑ **Part D**

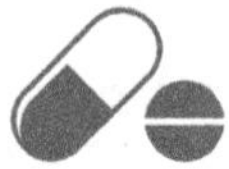

☑ **Some extra benefits**

Some plans also include:

☐ **Lower out-of-pocket costs**

See Section 4 (starting on page 61) to learn more about Medicare Advantage.

AT A GLANCE

Original Medicare vs. Medicare Advantage

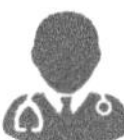 Doctor & hospital choice

Original Medicare	Medicare Advantage (Part C)
You can use **any doctor or hospital that takes Medicare, anywhere in the U.S.**	In many cases, you can only use **doctors and other providers who are in the plan's network and** service area (for non-emergency care). Some plans offer non-emergency coverage out of network, but typically at a higher cost.
In most cases, you **don't need** a referral to use a specialist.	You **may need** to get a referral to use a specialist.

 Cost

Original Medicare	Medicare Advantage (Part C)
For Part B-covered services, **you usually pay 20% of the** Medicare-approved **amount** after you meet your deductible. This amount is called your coinsurance.	**Out-of-pocket costs vary**—plans may have lower or higher out-of-pocket costs for certain services.
You **pay a** premium **(monthly payment) for Part B**. If you choose to join a Medicare drug plan, you'll pay a separate premium for your Medicare drug coverage (Part D).	You pay the monthly **Part B premium** and may also have to **pay the plan's premium**. Some plans may have a $0 premium and may help pay all or part of your Part B premium. Most plans include Medicare drug coverage (Part D).
There's **no yearly limit** on what you pay out of pocket, unless you have supplemental coverage—like Medicare Supplement Insurance (Medigap).	Plans **have a yearly limit** on what you pay out of pocket for services Medicare Part A and Part B cover. Once you reach your plan's limit, you'll pay nothing for services Part A and Part B cover for the rest of the year.
You **can get** Medigap to help pay your remaining out-of-pocket costs (like your 20% coinsurance). Or, you can use coverage from a former employer or union, or Medicaid.	You **can't buy and don't need** Medigap.

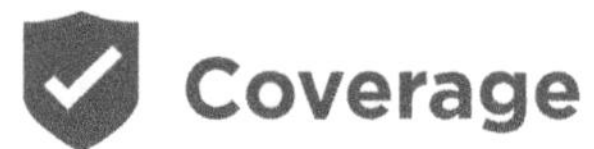

Coverage

Original Medicare	Medicare Advantage (Part C)
Original Medicare covers most medically necessary services and supplies in hospitals, doctors' offices, and other health care facilities. Original Medicare doesn't cover some benefits like eye exams, most dental care, and routine exams. See page 55.	Plans must cover all medically necessary services that Original Medicare covers. Plans may also offer some **extra benefits that Original Medicare doesn't cover**—like vision, hearing, and dental services.
You can join a **separate Medicare drug plan** to get Medicare drug coverage (Part D).	**Medicare drug coverage (Part D) is included in most plans.** In most types of Medicare Advantage Plans, you can't join a separate Medicare drug plan.
In most cases, you don't have to get a service or supply approved ahead of time for Original Medicare to cover it.	In many cases, you have to get a service or supply approved ahead of time for the plan to cover it.

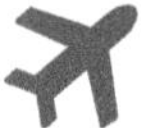

Foreign travel

Original Medicare	Medicare Advantage (Part C)
Original Medicare generally **doesn't cover medical care outside the U.S.** You may be able to buy a Medicare Supplement Insurance (Medigap) policy that covers emergency care outside the U.S.	Plans generally **don't cover medical care outside the U.S.** Some plans may offer a supplemental benefit that covers emergency and urgently needed services when traveling outside the U.S.

This handbook explains these topics in more detail:

- **Original Medicare:** See Section 3 (starting on page 57).
- **Medicare Advantage:** See Section 4 (starting on page 61).
- **Medicare Supplement Insurance (Medigap):** See Section 5 (starting on page 75).
- **Medicare drug coverage (Part D):** See Section 6 (starting on page 79).

Get started with Medicare

It's important for you to:

- **Understand your Medicare coverage options.** There are 2 main ways to get your Medicare coverage—Original Medicare (Part A and Part B) and Medicare Advantage. See pages 10–12 to learn more.
- **Find out how and when you can sign up.** If you don't have Medicare Part A or Part B, see Section 1 (starting on page 15). If you don't have Medicare drug coverage (Part D), see Section 6 (starting on page 79). **There may be penalties if you don't sign up when you're first eligible.** If you have other health insurance, see pages 19–22 to find out how your other insurance works with Medicare.
- **Mark your calendar with these important dates!** This may be the only chance you have each year to change your coverage.

October 1, 2022	**Start comparing your current coverage with other options.** You may be able to save money or get extra benefits. Visit Medicare.gov/plan-compare.
October 15 to December 7, 2022	**Change your Medicare health or drug coverage for 2023, if you decide to.** You can join, switch or drop a Medicare Advantage Plan or a Medicare drug plan during this Open Enrollment Period each year.
January 1, 2023	**New coverage begins if you made a change.** If you kept your existing coverage and your plan's costs or benefits changed, those changes also start on this date.
January 1 to March 31, 2023	**If you're in a Medicare Advantage Plan,** you can change to a different Medicare Advantage Plan or switch to Original Medicare (and join a separate Medicare drug plan) once during this time. Any changes you make will be effective the first of the month after the plan gets your request. See page 63.

Each year, it's important to review your Medicare health and drug coverage to see if it still meets your needs, and decide if you want to make a change. You don't need to sign up for Medicare each year, but you should still review your options.

See pages 10–14 for an overview of your Medicare options.

Get the most out of Medicare

Find a coverage option that's right for you

- Get free, personalized health insurance counseling from your State Health Insurance Assistance Program (SHIP). See pages 115–118 for the phone number of your local SHIP. A trusted agent or broker may also be able to help.
- Call 1-800-MEDICARE (1-800-633-4227). TTY users can call 1-877-486-2048.
- Find and compare health and drug plans at Medicare.gov/plan-compare.

Get the most value out of your health care

We want to make sure you have the information you need to make the best decisions about your health care. Look for throughout this handbook to learn about costs and coverage for services.

Learn about preventive services

Medicare covers many preventive services at no cost to you. Ask your doctor or other health care provider which preventive services (like screenings, shots or vaccines, and yearly "Wellness" visits) you need. See pages 30–55 and look for to learn more about which preventive services Medicare covers.

Get help paying for health care

There are multiple programs available to help with costs. Many people with Medicare qualify. For more on these programs, see pages 91–96.

Review your handbook online

Help Medicare save money by switching to the electronic version of this handbook. Log into (or create) your secure Medicare account at Medicare.gov to switch to the electronic handbook. We'll email you a link to a PDF version instead of sending a paper copy in the mail each fall.

SECTION 1

Signing up for Medicare

Will I get Part A and Part B automatically?

If you're already getting benefits from Social Security or the Railroad Retirement Board (RRB), you'll automatically get Part A and Part B starting the first day of the month you turn 65. (If your birthday is on the first day of the month, Part A and Part B starts the first day of the prior month.)

If you're under 65 and have a disability, you'll automatically get Part A and Part B after you get disability benefits from Social Security or certain disability benefits from the RRB for 24 months.

Remember, if you live in Puerto Rico, you don't automatically get Part B. You must sign up for it. See page 16.

If you have ALS (amyotrophic lateral sclerosis, also called Lou Gehrig's disease), you'll get Part A and Part B automatically the month your Social Security disability benefits begin.

If you automatically get Medicare, you'll get your red, white, and blue Medicare card in the mail 3 months before your 65th birthday or 25th month of disability benefits, and you don't need to pay a premium for Part A (sometimes called "premium-free Part A"). Most people choose to keep Part B. If you don't want Part B, let us know before the coverage start date on your Medicare card. If you do nothing, you'll keep Part B and will have to pay Part B premiums through your Social Security benefits. If you need help deciding if you should keep Part B, see page 19. **If you choose not to keep Part B but decide you want it later, you may have a delay in getting Medicare Part B coverage, and you may have to pay a late enrollment penalty for as long as you have Part B.** See page 23.

If you need to get a replacement Medicare card because it's damaged or lost, log into (or create) your secure Medicare account at Medicare.gov to print or order an official copy of your Medicare card. You can also call 1-800-MEDICARE (1-800-633-4227) to get a replacement card. TTY users can call 1-877-486-2048.

If you get Railroad Retirement Board (RRB) benefits, you can call 1-877-772-5772 to get a replacement card. TTY users can call 1-312-751-4701.

Will I have to sign up for Part A and/or Part B?

If you're close to 65, but NOT getting Social Security or Railroad Retirement Board (RRB) benefits, you'll need to sign up for Medicare. Visit ssa.gov/benefits/medicare to apply for Part A and Part B. You can also contact Social Security 3 months before you turn 65 to set up an appointment. If you worked for a railroad, contact the RRB.

In most cases, if you don't sign up for Part B when you're first eligible, you may have a delay in getting Medicare Part B coverage in the future, and **you may have to pay a late enrollment penalty for as long as you have Part B.** See page 23.

If you have End-Stage Renal Disease (ESRD) and you want Medicare, you'll need to sign up for it. Contact Social Security to find out when and how to sign up for Part A and Part B. For more information, visit Medicare.gov/publications to view the booklet, "Medicare Coverage of Kidney Dialysis & Kidney Transplant Services."

Important! **If you live in Puerto Rico and get benefits from Social Security or the RRB,** you'll automatically get Part A the first day of the month you turn 65 or after you get disability benefits for 24 months. However, if you want Part B, you'll need to sign up for it by completing an "Application for Enrollment in Part B Form" (CMS-40B). Visit Medicare.gov/basics/forms-publications-mailings/forms/enrollment to get Form CMS-40B in English or Spanish. If you don't sign up for Part B when you're first eligible, **you may have to pay a late enrollment penalty for as long as you have Part B.** See page 23.

Where can I get more information?

Call Social Security at 1-800-772-1213 for more information about your Medicare eligibility and to sign up for Part A and/or Part B. TTY users can call 1-800-325-0778. If you worked for a railroad or get RRB benefits, call the RRB at 1-877-772-5772. TTY users can call 1-312-751-4701.

You can also get free, personalized health insurance counseling from your State Health Insurance Assistance Program (SHIP). See pages 115–118 for the phone number of your local SHIP.

After you've signed up for Medicare Part A and/or Part B, it's time to look at your coverage options. People get Medicare coverage in different ways. To get the most out of your coverage, review all of your options and decide what best meets your needs. See pages 11–13 for more details.

If I didn't get Part A and Part B automatically, when can I sign up?

If you didn't automatically get **premium-free Part A** (for example, because you're still working and not yet getting Social Security or Railroad Retirement Board (RRB) benefits), you can sign up for it anytime after you're first eligible for Medicare. See page 22 for more information.

In this example, your Part A coverage will go back (retroactively) 6 months from when you sign up for Part A or apply for Social Security or RRB benefits, but no earlier than the first month you're eligible for Medicare. Depending on how you become eligible for Part A, the retroactive period may be different.

Note: You can only sign up for Part B during the enrollment periods listed below.

Important! **Remember, in most cases, if you don't sign up for Part A (if you have to buy it) and Part B when you're first eligible, your enrollment may be delayed and you may have to pay a late enrollment penalty. See pages 22–23.**

What are the Part A and Part B enrollment periods?

You can only sign up for Part B (and/or Part A if you have to buy it) during these enrollment periods.

Initial Enrollment Period

You can first sign up for Part A and/or Part B during the 7-month period that begins 3 months before the month you turn 65, includes the month you turn 65, and ends 3 months after the month you turn 65.

If you sign up for Part A and/or Part B during the first 3 months of your Initial Enrollment Period, in most cases, your coverage begins the first day of your birthday month. However, if your birthday is on the first day of the month, your coverage starts the first day of the prior month.

If you sign up and are paying for Part A and/or Part B the month you turn 65 or during the last 3 months of your Initial Enrollment Period, the start date for your Part B coverage will be delayed (in 2022).

New! If you sign up the month you turn 65 or during the last 3 months of your Initial Enrollment Period, your coverage starts the first day of the month after you sign up.

Special Enrollment Period

After your Initial Enrollment Period is over, you may have a chance to sign up for Medicare during a Special Enrollment Period. For example, if you didn't sign up for Part B (or Part A if you have to buy it) when you were first eligible because you have group health plan coverage based on current employment (your own, a spouse's, or a family member's if you have a disability), you can sign up for Part A and/or Part B:

- Anytime you're still covered by the group health plan
- During the 8-month period that begins the month after the employment ends or the coverage ends, whichever happens first

Usually, you won't have to pay a late enrollment penalty if you sign up during a Special Enrollment Period. This period doesn't apply if you're eligible for Medicare based on End-Stage Renal Disease (ESRD), or you're still in your Initial Enrollment Period.

Note: If you have a disability, and the group health plan coverage is based on a family member's current employment (other than a spouse), the employer offering the group health plan must have 100 or more employees for you to get a Special Enrollment Period.

Important! **COBRA (Consolidated Omnibus Budget Reconciliation Act) coverage, retiree health plans, VA coverage, and individual health insurance coverage (like coverage through the Health Insurance Marketplace®) aren't considered coverage based on current employment.** There may be reasons why you should take Part B instead of, or in addition to, COBRA coverage. You have 8 months after your coverage based on current employment ends to sign up for Part B without a penalty, whether or not you choose COBRA. However, if you have COBRA and you're eligible for Medicare, **COBRA may only pay a small portion of your medical costs.** You aren't eligible for a Special Enrollment Period to sign up for Medicare when that COBRA coverage ends. See page 88 for more information about COBRA coverage. To avoid paying a higher premium, make sure you sign up for Medicare when you're first eligible. If you have retiree coverage, it **may not** pay for your health services if you don't have both Part A and Part B.

New! There are other circumstances where you may be able to sign up for Medicare during a Special Enrollment Period. You may be eligible for a Special Enrollment Period if you miss an enrollment period because of certain exceptional circumstances, like being impacted by a natural disaster or an emergency, incarceration, employer or health plan error, or losing Medicaid coverage. For more information, visit Medicare.gov or call 1-800-MEDICARE (1-800-633-4227). TTY users can call 1-877-486-2048.

General Enrollment Period

If you have to pay for Part A but don't sign up for it and/or don't sign up for Part B (for which you must pay premiums) during your Initial Enrollment Period, and you don't qualify for a Special Enrollment Period, you can sign up during the General Enrollment Period from January 1–March 31 each year. **You may have to pay a higher Part A and/or Part B premium for late enrollment.** See pages 22–23.

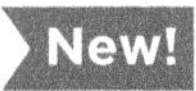

When you sign up during this period, your coverage starts the first day of the month after you sign up.

Not sure if you qualify for an enrollment period? Visit Medicare.gov or call 1-800-MEDICARE (1-800-633-4227). TTY users can call 1-877-486-2048.

I have other health coverage. Should I get Part B?

This information can help you decide if you should get Part B based on the type of health coverage you may have.

Employer or union coverage

If you or your spouse (or family member if you have a disability) **are still working** and you have health coverage through that employer or union, see page 21 to find out how your coverage works with Medicare. You can also contact the employer or union benefits administration for information. This includes federal or state employment and active-duty military service. It might be to your advantage to delay Part B enrollment while you still have health coverage based on your or your spouse's current employment.

Coverage based on current employment doesn't include:

- COBRA
- Retiree coverage
- VA coverage
- Individual health insurance coverage (like through the Health Insurance Marketplace®)

TRICARE

If you have TRICARE (health care program for active-duty and retired service members and their families), **you generally must sign up for Part A and Part B when you're first eligible to keep your TRICARE coverage.** However, if you're an active-duty service member or an active-duty family member, you don't have to sign up for Part B to keep your TRICARE coverage. For more information, contact your TRICARE contractor. See page 90.

If you have CHAMPVA coverage, you must sign up for Part A and Part B to keep it. Call 1-800-733-8387 for more information about CHAMPVA.

Medicaid

If you have Medicaid and don't have Part B, Medicaid may help you sign up for it. Medicare will pay first, and Medicaid will pay second. Medicaid may be able to help pay your Medicare out-of-pocket costs (like premiums, deductibles, coinsurance, and copayments).

Call your State Medical Assistance (Medicaid) office for more information and to find out if you qualify. Visit Medicare.gov/talk-to-someone, or call 1-800-MEDICARE (1-800-633-4227) to get the phone number for your state's Medicaid office.

Health Insurance Marketplace®

Even if you have Marketplace coverage, you should generally sign up for Medicare when you're first eligible to avoid the risk of a delay in Medicare coverage and the possibility of a Medicare late enrollment penalty.

Here are some important points to consider if you have Marketplace coverage:

- You need to end your Marketplace coverage in a timely manner when you become eligible for Medicare to avoid an overlap in coverage.
- Once you're considered eligible for Part A, or already have it, you won't qualify for help from the Marketplace to pay your Marketplace plan **premiums** or other medical costs. If you continue to get help paying for your Marketplace plan premiums after you have Medicare, you may have to pay back some or all of the help you got when you file your federal income taxes.

Visit **HealthCare.gov** to connect to the Marketplace in your state and learn more. To find out how to end your Marketplace plan or Marketplace savings when your Medicare coverage begins, visit **HealthCare.gov/medicare/changing-from-marketplace-to-medicare**. You can also call the Marketplace Call Center at 1-800-318-2596. TTY users can call 1-855-889-4325.

Health Savings Account (HSA)

You aren't eligible to make contributions to an HSA after you have Medicare. To avoid a tax penalty, you should make your last HSA contribution the month before your Part A coverage begins. Premium-free Part A coverage will go back (retroactively) 6 months from when you sign up for Part A or apply for benefits from Social Security or the Railroad Retirement Board, but no earlier than the first month you're eligible for Medicare. Depending on how you become eligible for Part A, the retroactive period may be different. See the chart below to help decide when it's best to stop your HSA contributions.

If you sign up for Medicare:	During your Initial Enrollment Period	You can avoid a tax penalty by making your last HSA contribution the month before you turn 65.
	2 months after your Initial Enrollment Period ends	
If you wait to sign up for Medicare:	Less than 6 months after you turn 65	You can avoid a tax penalty by stopping HSA contributions the month before you turn 65.
	6 or more months after you turn 65	You can avoid a tax penalty by stopping HSA contributions 6 months before the month you apply for Medicare.

Note: A Medicare Medical Savings Account (MSA) plan is similar to an HSA plan. See page 67.

How does my other insurance work with Medicare?

When you have other insurance (like group health plan, retiree health, or Medicaid coverage) and Medicare, there are rules for whether Medicare or your other coverage pays first.

If you have **retiree** health coverage (like insurance from your or your spouse's former employment)...	Medicare pays first.
If you're 65 or older, have group health plan coverage based on your or your spouse's **current** employment, and the employer has **20 or more employees**...	Your group health plan pays first.
If you're 65 or older, have group health plan coverage based on your or your spouse's **current** employment, and the employer has **fewer than 20 employees**...	Medicare pays first.
If you're under 65 and have a disability, have group health plan coverage based on your or a family member's **current** employment, and the employer has **100 or more employees**...	Your group health plan pays first.
If you're under 65 and have a disability, have group health plan coverage based on your or a family member's **current** employment, and the employer has **fewer than 100 employees**...	Medicare pays first.
If you have group health plan coverage based on your or a family member's employment or former employment, and you're eligible for Medicare because of End-Stage Renal Disease (ESRD)...	Your group health plan pays first for the first 30 months after you become eligible for Medicare. Medicare pays first after this 30-month period.
If you have TRICARE...	Medicare pays first, unless you're on active duty, or get items or services from a military hospital or clinic, or other federal health care provider.
If you have Medicaid...	Medicare pays first.

Important! If you're still working and have employer coverage through work, contact your employer to find out how your employer's coverage works with Medicare.

Here are some important facts to remember about how other insurance works with Medicare-covered services:

- The insurance that pays first (primary payer) pays up to the limits of its coverage.
- The insurance that pays second (secondary payer) only pays if there are costs the primary payer didn't cover.
- The secondary payer (which may be Medicare) might not pay all of the uncovered costs.
- If your group health plan or retiree health coverage is the secondary payer, you might need to sign up for Part B before your insurance will pay.

Visit Medicare.gov/publications to view the booklet, "Medicare and Other Health Benefits: Your Guide to Who Pays First." You can also call 1-800-MEDICARE (1-800-633-4227) for more information. TTY users can call 1-877-486-2048.

Important! If you have other insurance or changes to your insurance, you need to let Medicare know by calling Medicare's Benefits Coordination & Recovery Center at 1-855-798-2627. TTY users can call 1-855-797-2627.

If you have Part A, you may get a "Health Coverage" form (IRS Form 1095-B) from Medicare. This form verifies that you had health coverage in the past year. Keep the form for your records. Not everyone will get this form. If you don't get Form 1095-B, don't worry. You don't need it to file your taxes.

Do I have to pay for Part A?

You usually don't pay a monthly premium for Part A coverage if you or your spouse paid Medicare taxes while working for a certain amount of time. This is sometimes called premium-free Part A. If you aren't eligible for premium-free Part A, you may be able to buy it. For more information on how to pay your Part A premium, see page 24.

If you buy Part A, you'll pay a premium of either $278 or up to $506 each month in 2023 depending on how long you or your spouse worked and paid Medicare taxes. If you need help paying your Part A premium, see pages 94–96. If you have questions about paying for Part A, visit Medicare.gov or call 1-800-MEDICARE (1-800-633-4227). TTY users can call 1-877-486-2048.

In most cases, if you choose to **buy** Part A, you must also have Part B and pay monthly premiums for both. If you choose NOT to buy Part A, you can still buy Part B if you're eligible.

What's the Part A late enrollment penalty?

If you aren't eligible for premium-free Part A, and you don't buy it when you're first eligible, your monthly premium may go up 10%. You'll have to pay the higher premium for twice the number of years you could have had Part A but didn't sign up. For example, if you were eligible for Part A for 2 years but didn't sign up, you'll have to pay a 10% higher premium for 4 years.

How much does Part B coverage cost?

The standard Part B premium amount in 2023 is $164.90. Most people pay the standard Part B premium amount every month.

If your modified adjusted gross income is above a certain amount (in 2023: $97,000 if you file individually or $194,000 if you're married and file jointly), you may pay an Income Related Monthly Adjustment Amount (IRMAA). IRMAA is an extra charge added to your premium.

To determine if you'll pay the IRMAA, Medicare uses the modified adjusted gross income reported on your IRS tax return from 2 years ago. Visit Medicare.gov to learn more about IRMAA determinations.

Note: You may also pay an extra amount for your Medicare drug coverage (Part D) premium if your modified adjusted gross income is above a certain amount. See page 82.

If you have to pay an extra amount and you disagree (for example, your income is lower due to a life event), visit ssa.gov or call Social Security at 1-800-772-1213. TTY users can call 1-800-325-0778.

What's the Part B late enrollment penalty?

Important! **If you don't sign up for Part B when you're first eligible, you may have to pay a late enrollment penalty for as long as you have Part B.** Your monthly Part B premium may go up 10% for each full 12 months in the period that you could've had Part B, but didn't sign up. If you're allowed to sign up for Part B during a Special Enrollment Period, you usually don't pay a late enrollment penalty. See pages 17–18.

Example: Mr. Smith's Initial Enrollment Period ended December 2019. He waited until March 2022 (during the General Enrollment Period) to sign up for Part B. His Part B premium penalty is 20%, and he'll have to pay this penalty in addition to his standard Part B premium for as long as he has Part B. (Even though Mr. Smith wasn't covered a total of 27 months, this included only 2 full 12-month periods.)

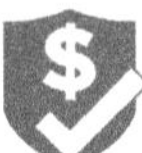

Cost & coverage: To learn how to get help with Medicare costs, see Section 7 (starting on page 91).

How can I pay my Part B premium?

If you get Social Security or Railroad Retirement Board (RRB) benefits, your Part B premium will be deducted from your monthly benefit payment.

If you're a federal retiree with an annuity from the Office of Personnel Management and not entitled to Social Security or RRB benefits, you may request to have your Part B premiums deducted from your annuity. Call 1-800-MEDICARE (1-800-633-4227) to make your request. TTY users can call 1-877-486-2048.

If you don't get these benefit payments, you'll get a bill for your Part B premium. Typically, Part B premiums are billed quarterly (every 3 months). If you also pay for Part A or Part D IRMAA, or enroll in Medicare Easy Pay to pay your premiums, you'll get a monthly bill (see pages 22 and 82). There are 4 ways to pay your premium bill:

1. **Pay online by credit card, debit card, savings or checking account.** To do this, log into (or create) your secure Medicare account at Medicare.gov. Paying online is a more secure and faster way to make your payment without sending your personal information in the mail. You'll get a confirmation number when you make your payment.
2. **Pay directly from your savings or checking account through your bank's online bill payment services.** Ask your bank if it allows customers to pay bills online—not all banks offer this service and some may charge a fee. Your bank will need this information:
   - **Your Medicare Number:** It's important that you **use the exact number** on your red, white, and blue Medicare card, but without the dashes.
   - **Payee name:** CMS Medicare Insurance
   - **Payee address:**
     Medicare Premium Collection Center
     PO Box 790355
     St. Louis, MO 63179-0355
3. **Sign up for Medicare Easy Pay.** This is a free service that automatically deducts your premium payments from your savings or checking account each month. Visit Medicare.gov/medicare-easy-pay, or call 1-800-MEDICARE (1-800-633-4227) to find out how to sign up. TTY users can call 1-877-486-2048.
4. **Mail your payment to Medicare.** You can pay by check, money order, credit card, or debit card. Write your Medicare Number on your payment, and fill out your payment coupon. Mail your payment and coupon to:

   Medicare Premium Collection Center
   PO Box 790355
   St. Louis, MO 63179-0355

If you have questions about your premiums, call 1-800-MEDICARE or visit Medicare.gov.

If you need to change your address on your bill, call Social Security at 1-800-772-1213. TTY users can call 1-800-325-0778.

Note to RRB Annuitants: If you get a bill from the RRB, mail your premium payments to:

RRB Medicare Premium Payments
PO Box 979024
St. Louis, MO 63197-9000

If your bills are from the RRB, call 1-877-772-5772. TTY users can call 1-312-751-4701.

Important! **Need help paying for your Part B premium?** See pages 94–95.

SECTION 2

Find out if Medicare covers your test, item, or service

What services does Medicare cover?

Medicare Part A and Part B cover certain medical services and supplies in hospitals, doctors' offices, and other health care facilities. Medicare Part D covers prescription drugs.

Your red, white, and blue Medicare card shows whether you have Part A (listed as HOSPITAL), Part B (listed as MEDICAL), or both, and the date your coverage begins. If you have Original Medicare, you'll use it to get your Medicare-covered services. If you join a Medicare Advantage Plan or other Medicare health plan, in most cases, you'll use your plan's card to get your Medicare-covered services.

You can get all of the Medicare-covered services in this section if you have both Part A and Part B.

Note: If you're not lawfully present in the U.S., Medicare won't pay for your Part A and Part B claims, and you can't join a Medicare Advantage Plan or a Medicare drug plan.

What does Part A cover?

Part A (Hospital Insurance) helps cover:

- Inpatient care in a hospital
- Inpatient care in a skilled nursing facility **(not custodial or long-term care)**
- Hospice care
- Home health care
- Inpatient care in a religious non-medical health care institution

See pages 26–29 for a list of common services Part A covers and general descriptions.

For more information on Part A-covered services, visit Medicare.gov/coverage.

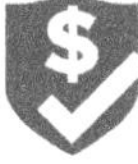

Cost & coverage: **Find out what's covered using your mobile device**
To get Medicare coverage information, download Medicare's free "What's covered" mobile app on your smartphone or tablet. "What's covered" is available in the App Store and on Google Play.

Note: See pages 119–122 for definitions of blue words.

What do I pay for Part A-covered services?

Copayments, coinsurance, or deductibles may apply for each service listed on the following pages.

If you're in a Medicare Advantage Plan or have other insurance (like Medigap, Medicaid, or employer or union coverage), your copayments, coinsurance, or deductibles may be different. For more information about costs, contact your plan or visit

 Medicare.gov/plan-compare.

You can also call 1-800-MEDICARE (1-800-633-4227). TTY users can call 1-877-486-2048.

Part A-covered services

Blood

If the hospital gets blood from a blood bank at no charge, you won't have to pay for it or replace it. If the hospital has to buy blood for you, you must either pay the hospital costs for the first 3 units of blood you get in a calendar year, or you or someone else can donate the blood.

Home health services

Part A and/or Part B covers home health benefits. See page 44.

Hospice care

To qualify for hospice care, a hospice doctor and your doctor (if you have one) must certify that you're terminally ill, meaning you have a life expectancy of 6 months or less. When you agree to hospice care, you're agreeing to comfort care (palliative care) instead of care to cure your terminal illness. You also must sign a statement choosing hospice care instead of other Medicare-covered treatments for your terminal illness and related conditions.

Coverage includes:

- All items and services needed for pain relief and symptom management
- Medical, nursing, and social services
- Drugs for pain and symptom management
- Durable medical equipment for pain relief and symptom management
- Aide and homemaker services
- Other covered services you need to manage your pain and other symptoms, as well as spiritual and grief counseling for you and your family

Medicare-certified hospice care is usually given in your home or other facility where you live, like a nursing home. Original Medicare will still pay for covered benefits for any health problems that aren't part of your terminal illness and related conditions, but hospice should cover most of your care.

Medicare won't pay room and board for your care in a facility unless the hospice medical team decides you need short-term inpatient care to manage pain and other symptoms. This care must be in a Medicare-approved facility, like a hospice facility, hospital, or skilled nursing facility that contracts with the hospice.

Medicare also covers inpatient respite care, which is care you get in a Medicare-approved facility so that your usual caregiver (family member or friend) can rest. You can stay up to 5 days each time you get respite care.

After 6 months, you can continue to get hospice care as long as the hospice medical director or hospice doctor recertifies (at a face-to-face meeting) that you're still terminally ill.

You pay:
- Nothing for hospice care.
- A copayment of up to $5 per prescription for outpatient drugs for pain and symptom management.
- Five percent of the Medicare-approved amount for inpatient respite care.

Original Medicare will be billed for your hospice care, even if you're in a Medicare Advantage Plan. When you get hospice care, your Medicare Advantage Plan can still cover services that aren't a part of your terminal illness or any conditions related to your terminal illness. Contact your plan for more information.

Inpatient hospital care

Medicare covers semi-private rooms, meals, general nursing, drugs (including methadone to treat an opioid use disorder), and other hospital services and supplies as part of your inpatient treatment. This includes care you get in acute care hospitals, critical access hospitals, inpatient rehabilitation facilities, long-term care hospitals, psychiatric care in inpatient psychiatric facilities, and inpatient care for a qualifying clinical research study. This doesn't include private-duty nursing, a television or phone in your room (if there's a separate charge for these items), personal care items (razors or slipper socks), or a private room, unless medically necessary.

If you also have Part B, it generally covers 80% of the Medicare-approved amount for doctors' services you get while you're in a hospital.

In each benefit period, you pay:
- **Days 1–60:** Nothing after you meet your Part A deductible.
- **Days 61–90:** A $400 copayment each day.
- **Days 91–150:** A $800 copayment each day while using your 60 lifetime reserve days.
- **After day 150:** You pay all costs after you use all of your lifetime reserve days.

You can only get inpatient psychiatric care in a freestanding psychiatric hospital 190 days in a lifetime.

Note: Hospitals are now required to make public the standard charges for all of their items and services (including the standard charges negotiated by Medicare Advantage Plans) to help you make more informed decisions about your care.

Am I an inpatient or outpatient?

Whether you're an inpatient or an outpatient affects how much you pay for hospital services and if you qualify for Part A skilled nursing facility care.

- You're an inpatient when the hospital formally admits you with a doctor's order.
- You're an outpatient if you're getting emergency or observation services (which may include an overnight stay in the hospital or services in an outpatient clinic), lab tests, or X-rays, without a formal inpatient admission (even if you spend the night in the hospital).

Each day you have to stay, you or your caregiver should always ask the hospital and/or your doctor, or a hospital social worker or patient advocate, if you're an inpatient or outpatient.

Sometimes doctors will keep you as an outpatient for observation services while they decide whether to admit you as an inpatient or release (discharge) you. If you're under observation more than 24 hours, you must get a "Medicare Outpatient Observation Notice" (also called "MOON"). This notice tells you why you're an outpatient (in a hospital or critical access hospital) getting observation services, and how it affects what you pay in the hospital and for care after you leave.

Religious non-medical health care institution (inpatient care)

If you qualify for inpatient hospital or skilled nursing facility care in these facilities, Medicare will only cover inpatient, non-religious, non-medical items and services, like room and board, and items or services that don't need a doctor's order or prescription (like unmedicated wound dressings or use of a simple walker). Medicare doesn't cover the religious portion of this type of care.

Skilled nursing facility care

Medicare covers semi-private rooms, meals, skilled nursing and therapy services, and other medically necessary services and supplies in a skilled nursing facility. **Medicare only covers these services after a 3-day minimum medically necessary inpatient hospital stay** (not including the day you leave the hospital) for an illness or injury related to the hospital stay. If you're in a Medicare Advantage Plan, you may not need a 3-day hospital stay. Check with your plan.

Note: You may not need a 3-day minimum inpatient hospital stay if your doctor participates in an Accountable Care Organization or an entity participating in another type of Medicare initiative approved for a Skilled Nursing Facility 3-Day Rule Waiver. See pages 111–112.

You may get skilled nursing care or therapy if it's necessary to improve or maintain your current condition. You can appeal if you disagree with your discharge, like if the discharge is based solely on a lack of improvement, even though you still require skilled nursing or therapy care to keep your condition from getting worse. See page 100 for more information about your rights to appeal.

To qualify for skilled nursing facility care, your doctor must certify that you need daily skilled care (like intravenous fluids/medications or physical therapy) which, as a practical matter, you can only get as a skilled nursing facility inpatient. Medicare doesn't cover non-medical long-term care. See page 56.

You pay:

- Nothing for the first 20 days of each benefit period.
  Note: If you're in a Medicare Advantage Plan, you may be charged copayments during the first 20 days.
- A coinsurance amount per day for days 21–100 of each benefit period.
- All costs for each day after day 100 in a benefit period.

What does Part B cover?

Medicare Part B (Medical Insurance) helps cover medically necessary doctor's services, outpatient care, home health services, durable medical equipment, mental health services, and other medical services. Part B also covers many preventive services. See pages 30–55 for a list of common Part B-covered services and general descriptions. Medicare may cover some services and tests more often than the timeframes listed if needed to diagnose or treat a condition. To find out if Medicare covers a service that isn't on this list or for more on Part-B covered services, visit

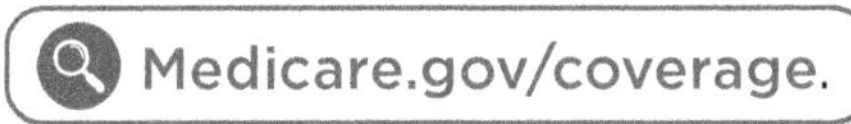
Medicare.gov/coverage.

Or, call 1-800-MEDICARE (1-800-633-4227). TTY users can call 1-877-486-2048.

What do I pay for services Part B covers?

The list of covered services (in alphabetical order on the following pages) gives general information about what you pay if you have Original Medicare and see doctors or other health care providers who accept assignment (see page 59). You'll pay more if you see doctors or providers who don't accept assignment. **If you're in a Medicare Advantage Plan or have other insurance (like Medigap, Medicaid, or employer or union coverage), your copayments, coinsurance, or deductibles may be different.** Contact your plan for more information.

Under Original Medicare, if the Part B deductible applies, you must pay all costs (up to the Medicare-approved amount) until you meet the yearly Part B deductible. After you meet your deductible, Medicare begins to pay its share and you typically pay 20% of the Medicare-approved amount of the service (if the doctor or other health care provider accepts assignment). **There's no yearly limit on what you pay out of pocket if you have Original Medicare.** There may be limits on expenses you pay through supplemental coverage you may have, like Medigap, Medicaid, or employer or union coverage.

You pay nothing for most covered preventive services if you get the services from a doctor or other qualified health care provider who accepts assignment. However, for some preventive services, you may have to pay a deductible, coinsurance, or both. These costs may also apply if you get a preventive service in the same visit as a non-preventive service.

Part B-covered services

You'll see this apple next to the preventive services on pages 30–55.

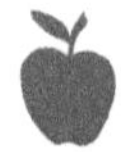

Preventive service

Abdominal aortic aneurysm screenings

Medicare covers an abdominal aortic aneurysm screening ultrasound once if you're at risk (only with a referral from your doctor or other qualified health care provider). You pay nothing for the screening if your doctor or other qualified health care provider accepts assignment.

Note: If you have a family history of abdominal aortic aneurysms, or you're a man 65–75 and have smoked at least 100 cigarettes in your lifetime, you're considered at risk.

Acupuncture

Medicare covers up to 12 acupuncture visits in 90 days for chronic low back pain defined as:

- Lasting 12 weeks or longer
- Not having an identifiable cause (for example, not an identifiable disease like cancer that has spread, or an infectious or inflammatory disease)
- Pain that isn't associated with surgery or pregnancy

Medicare covers an additional 8 sessions if you show improvement. If you aren't showing improvement, Medicare won't cover your additional treatments and they should be discontinued. You can get a maximum of 20 acupuncture treatments in a 12-month period. The Part B deductible and coinsurance apply.

Note: Not all providers can give acupuncture. Medicare doesn't cover acupuncture (including dry needling) for any condition other than chronic low back pain.

Advance care planning

Medicare covers voluntary advance care planning as part of your yearly "Wellness" visit (see page 55). This is planning for care you would get if you become unable to speak for yourself. As part of advance care planning, you may choose to complete an advance directive. This is an important legal document that records your wishes about medical treatment at a future time, if you aren't able to make decisions about your care. You can talk about an advance directive with your health care provider, and they can help you fill out the forms, if you prefer.

Consider carefully who you want to speak for you and what directions you want to give. You have the right to carry out your plans as you choose without discrimination based on your age or disability. You can update your advance directive at any time. You pay nothing if it's provided as part of the yearly "Wellness" visit, and your doctor or other qualified health care provider accepts assignment.

Note: Medicare may also cover this service as part of your medical treatment. When advance care planning isn't part of your yearly "Wellness" visit, the Part B deductible and coinsurance apply.

Need help with your advance directive? Visit the Eldercare Locator at eldercare.acl.gov to find help in your community.

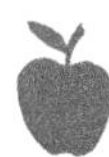

Preventive service

Alcohol misuse screenings & counseling

Medicare covers an alcohol misuse screening for adults (including pregnant individuals) who use alcohol, but don't meet the medical criteria for alcohol dependency. If your primary care doctor or other primary care provider determines you're misusing alcohol, you can get up to 4 brief, face-to-face counseling sessions per year (if you're competent and alert during counseling). You must get counseling in a primary care setting, like a doctor's office. You pay nothing if your qualified primary care doctor or other primary care provider accepts assignment.

Ambulance services

Medicare covers ground ambulance transportation to a hospital, critical access hospital, or skilled nursing facility for medically necessary services when traveling in any other vehicle could endanger your health. Medicare may pay for emergency ambulance transportation in an airplane or helicopter if you need immediate and rapid ambulance transport that ground transportation can't provide.

In some cases, Medicare may pay for limited, medically necessary, non-emergency ambulance transportation if you have a written order from your doctor stating that ambulance transportation is medically necessary. For example, someone with End-Stage Renal Disease (ESRD) may need a medically necessary ambulance transport to a facility that furnishes renal dialysis.

Medicare will only cover ambulance services to the nearest appropriate medical facility that's able to give you the care you need.

You pay 20% of the Medicare-approved amount. The Part B deductible applies.

Ambulatory surgical centers

Medicare covers the facility service fees related to approved surgical procedures provided in an ambulatory surgical center (outpatient facility where surgical procedures are performed, and the patient is expected to be released within 24 hours). Except for certain preventive services (for which you pay nothing if your doctor or other health care provider accepts assignment), you pay 20% of the Medicare-approved amount to both the ambulatory surgical center and the doctor who treats you. The Part B deductible applies. You pay all of the facility service fees for procedures Medicare doesn't cover in ambulatory surgical centers.

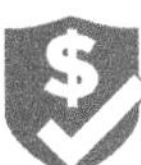

Cost & coverage: To get cost estimates for ambulatory surgical center outpatient procedures, visit

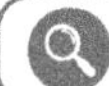 Medicare.gov/procedure-price-lookup.

Bariatric surgery

Medicare covers some bariatric surgical procedures, like gastric bypass surgery and laparoscopic banding surgery, when you meet certain conditions related to morbid obesity. For information on costs, visit **Medicare.gov/coverage/bariatric-surgery**.

Behavioral health integration services

If you have a behavioral health condition (like depression, anxiety, or another mental health condition), Medicare may pay your provider to help manage that condition. Some providers that manage behavioral health conditions may offer integrated care services, like the Psychiatric Collaborative Care Model. This model is a set of integrated behavioral health services, including care management support that may include:

- Care planning for behavioral health conditions
- Ongoing assessment of your condition
- Medication support
- Counseling
- Other treatment your provider recommends

Your health care provider will ask you to sign an agreement for you to get this set of services on a monthly basis. Your Part B **deductible** and **coinsurance** will apply to the monthly service fee.

Blood

If the provider gets blood from a blood bank at no charge, you won't have to pay for it or replace it. However, you'll pay a **copayment** for the blood processing and handling services for each unit of blood you get. The Part B deductible applies. If the provider has to buy blood for you, you must either pay the provider costs for the first 3 units of blood you get in a calendar year, or you or someone else can donate the blood.

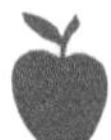

Preventive service

Bone mass measurements

This test helps to see if you're at risk for broken bones. Medicare covers it once every 24 months (more often if **medically necessary**) for people who have certain medical conditions or meet certain criteria. You pay nothing for this test if your doctor or other qualified health care provider accepts **assignment**.

Cardiac rehabilitation

Medicare covers comprehensive programs that include exercise, education, and counseling if you've had at least one of these conditions:

- A heart attack in the last 12 months
- Coronary artery bypass surgery
- Current stable angina pectoris (chest pain)
- A heart valve repair or replacement
- A coronary angioplasty (a medical procedure used to open a blocked artery) or coronary stenting (a procedure used to keep an artery open)
- A heart or heart-lung transplant
- Stable chronic heart failure

Medicare also covers intensive cardiac rehabilitation programs that are usually more rigorous or more intense than regular cardiac rehabilitation programs. Medicare covers services in a doctor's office or hospital outpatient setting. You pay 20% of the Medicare-approved amount if you get the services in a doctor's office, and a copayment in a hospital outpatient setting. The Part B deductible applies.

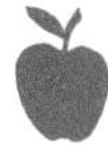

Preventive service

Cardiovascular behavioral therapy

Medicare covers a cardiovascular behavioral therapy visit one time each year with your primary care doctor or other qualified primary care provider in a primary care setting (like a doctor's office) to help lower your risk for cardiovascular disease. During this visit, your doctor may discuss aspirin use (if appropriate), check your blood pressure, and give you tips on eating well. You pay nothing if your primary care provider accepts assignment.

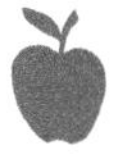

Preventive service

Cardiovascular disease screenings

These screenings include blood tests for cholesterol, lipid, and triglyceride levels that help detect conditions that may lead to a heart attack or stroke. Medicare covers these screening blood tests once every 5 years. You pay nothing for the tests if the doctor or other qualified health care provider accepts assignment.

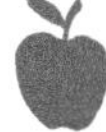

Preventive service

Cervical & vaginal cancer screenings

Medicare covers Pap tests and pelvic exams to check for cervical and vaginal cancers. As part of the pelvic exam, Medicare also covers a clinical breast exam to check for breast cancer. Medicare covers these screening tests once every 24 months in most cases. Medicare covers these screening tests once every 12 months if you're at high risk for cervical or vaginal cancer, or if you're of child-bearing age and had an abnormal Pap test in the past 36 months.

Medicare also covers Human Papillomavirus (HPV) tests (as part of a Pap test) once every 5 years if you're 30–65 without HPV symptoms.

You pay nothing for the lab Pap test, the lab HPV with the Pap test, the Pap test specimen collection, and pelvic and breast exams if your doctor or other qualified health care provider accepts assignment.

Chemotherapy

Medicare covers chemotherapy in a doctor's office, freestanding clinic, or hospital outpatient setting if you have cancer. You pay a copayment for chemotherapy in a hospital outpatient setting.

You pay 20% of the Medicare-approved amount for chemotherapy in a doctor's office or freestanding clinic. The Part B deductible applies.

For chemotherapy in an inpatient hospital setting covered under Part A, see inpatient hospital care on pages 27–28.

Chiropractic services

Medicare covers manipulation of the spine by a chiropractor to correct a subluxation (when the spinal joints fail to move properly, but the contact between the joints remains intact). You pay 20% of the Medicare-approved amount. The Part B deductible applies.

Note: Medicare doesn't cover other services or tests a chiropractor orders, other than manipulation of the spine.

Chronic care management services

If you have 2 or more serious chronic conditions (like arthritis and diabetes) that you expect to last at least a year, Medicare may pay for a health care provider's help to manage those conditions. This includes a comprehensive care plan that lists your health problems and goals, other providers, medications, community services you have and need, and other health information. It also explains the care you need and how it will be coordinated.

If you agree to get this service, your provider will prepare the care plan for you or your caregiver, help you with medication management, provide 24/7 access for urgent care management needs, give you support when you go from one health care setting to another, review your medicines and how you take them, and help you with other chronic care needs.

Note: You pay a monthly fee, and the Part B deductible and coinsurance apply. If you have supplemental insurance, including Medicaid, it may help cover the monthly fee.

Clinical research studies

Clinical research studies test how well different types of medical care work and if they're safe, like how well a cancer drug works. Medicare covers some costs, like office visits and tests in certain qualifying clinical research studies. You may pay 20% of the Medicare-approved amount, depending on the treatment you get. The Part B deductible may apply. Visit Medicare.gov/coverage/clinical-research-studies for more information.

Note: If you're in a Medicare Advantage Plan, Original Medicare may cover some costs along with your Medicare Advantage Plan.

Cognitive assessment & care plan services

When you see your provider for a visit (including your yearly "Wellness" visit), they may perform a cognitive assessment to look for signs of dementia, including Alzheimer's disease. Signs of cognitive impairment include trouble remembering, learning new things, concentrating, managing finances, or making decisions about your everyday life. Conditions like depression, anxiety, and delirium can also cause confusion, so it's important to understand why you may be having symptoms.

Medicare covers a separate visit with your regular doctor or a specialist to do a full review of your cognitive function, establish or confirm a diagnosis like dementia or Alzheimer's disease, and develop a care plan. You can bring someone with you, like a spouse, friend, or caregiver, to help provide information and answer questions.

During this visit, your doctor may:

- Perform an exam, talk with you about your medical history, and review your medications.
- Create a care plan to help address and manage your symptoms.
- Help you develop or update your advance care plan. See page 30.
- Refer you to a specialist, if needed.
- Help you understand more about community resources, like rehabilitation services, adult day health programs, and support groups.

The Part B deductible and coinsurance apply.

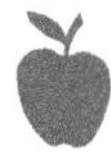

Preventive service

Colorectal cancer screenings

Medicare covers these screenings to help find precancerous growths or find cancer early, when treatment is most effective. Medicare may cover one or more of these screening tests:

- **Barium enema:** Medicare covers this test once every 48 months if you're 45 or older (or every 24 months if you're high risk) when your doctor uses it instead of a flexible sigmoidoscopy or colonoscopy. You pay 20% of the Medicare-approved amount for your doctors' services. In a hospital outpatient setting, you also pay the hospital a copayment. The Part B deductible doesn't apply.

  Visit Medicare.gov/coverage/barium-enemas for more information.
- **Colonoscopies:** Medicare covers this screening test once every 120 months (or every 24 months if you're high risk) or 48 months after a previous flexible sigmoidoscopy. There's no minimum age requirement. If you initially have a non-invasive stool-based screening test (fecal occult blood tests or multi-target stool DNA test) and receive a positive result, Medicare also covers a follow-up colonoscopy as a screening test. You pay nothing for the screening test(s) if your doctor or other qualified health care provider accepts assignment.
- **Flexible sigmoidoscopies:** Medicare covers this test once every 48 months if you're 45 or older, or 120 months after a previous screening colonoscopy if you aren't at high risk. You pay nothing for the test if your doctor or other qualified health care provider accepts assignment.

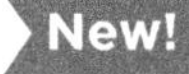

Note: If your doctor finds and removes a polyp or other tissue during the colonoscopy or flexible sigmoidoscopy, you pay 15% of the Medicare-approved amount for your doctors' services. In a hospital outpatient setting, you also pay the hospital a 15% coinsurance. The Part B deductible doesn't apply.

- **Fecal occult blood tests:** Medicare covers this test once every 12 months if you're 45 or older. You pay nothing for the test if your doctor or other qualified health care provider accepts assignment.

- **Multi-target stool DNA & blood-based biomarker tests:** Medicare covers these tests once every 3 years if you meet all of these conditions:
  - You're between 45–85.
  - You show no symptoms of colorectal disease including, but not limited to, lower gastrointestinal pain, blood in stool, a positive guaiac fecal occult blood test or fecal immunochemical test.
  - You're at average risk for developing colorectal cancer, meaning:
    - You have no personal history of adenomatous polyps, colorectal cancer, or inflammatory bowel disease, including Crohn's Disease and ulcerative colitis.
    - You have no family history of colorectal cancer or adenomatous polyps, familial adenomatous polyposis, or hereditary nonpolyposis colorectal cancer.

  Note: Multi-target stool DNA tests are at-home lab tests. Blood-based biomarker tests are conducted in a lab. You pay nothing for these tests if your doctor or other qualified health care provider accepts **assignment**.

Continuous Positive Airway Pressure (CPAP) devices, accessories, & therapy

Medicare may cover a 3-month trial of CPAP therapy (including devices and accessories) if you've been diagnosed with obstructive sleep apnea. After the trial period, Medicare may continue to cover CPAP therapy, devices and accessories if you meet with your doctor in person, and your doctor documents in your medical record that you meet certain conditions and the therapy is helping you.

You pay 20% of the **Medicare-approved amount** for the machine rental and purchase of related supplies (like masks and tubing). The Part B **deductible** applies. Medicare pays the supplier to rent the machine for 13 months if you've been using it without interruption. After you've rented the machine for 13 months, you own it.

Note: Medicare may cover rental or a replacement CPAP machine and/or CPAP accessories if you had a CPAP machine before you got Medicare, and you meet certain requirements.

Preventive service

Counseling to prevent tobacco use & tobacco-caused disease

Medicare covers up to 8 face-to-face visits in a 12-month period if you use tobacco. You pay nothing for the counseling sessions if your doctor or other qualified health care provider accepts assignment.

COVID-19 (Coronavirus disease 2019)

Your health and safety are our highest priority in the face of the coronavirus disease 2019 (COVID-19) public health emergency. Many people with Medicare are at higher risk for serious COVID-19 illness, so it's important to take the necessary steps to keep yourself and others safe.

Medicare covers several tests, items, and services related to COVID-19. Coverage could change when the public health emergency ends. Talk with your doctor or health care provider to see which are right for you:

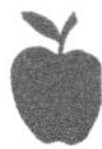

Preventive service

Vaccines:

- FDA-approved and FDA-authorized vaccines help reduce the risk of illness from COVID-19 by working with the body's natural defenses to safely develop immunity (protection) against the virus.
- You pay nothing for the COVID-19 vaccine if your doctor or other health care provider accepts **assignment** for giving the shot.
- Be sure to bring your red, white, and blue Medicare card with you when you get the vaccine so your health care provider or pharmacy can bill Medicare. If you're in a **Medicare Advantage Plan**, you must use the card from your plan to get your Medicare-covered services.

Diagnostic tests:

- These FDA-authorized tests check to see if you have COVID-19.
- You pay nothing when a health care provider orders this test during the COVID-19 public health emergency and you get it from a laboratory, pharmacy, doctor, or hospital.

Antibody tests:

- These FDA-authorized tests help see if you've developed an immune response and may not be at immediate risk of COVID-19 reinfection.
- You pay nothing for the test during the COVID-19 public health emergency.

Monoclonal antibody treatments and products:

- These FDA-authorized treatments can help fight the disease and keep you out of the hospital, if you test positive for COVID-19 and have mild to moderate symptoms.
- You pay nothing for this treatment during the COVID-19 public health emergency (and for the rest of the calendar year in which the Emergency Use Authorization (EUA) for this treatment ends) when you get it from a Medicare provider or supplier. You must meet certain conditions to qualify.
- In the calendar year after the EUA ends, Original Medicare will cover monoclonal antibody treatments if you have COVID-19 symptoms.

  Note: Certain monoclonal antibody products can protect you before you're exposed to COVID-19. If you have Part B and your doctor decides this type of product could work for you (like if you have a weakened immune system), you pay nothing for the product during or after the COVID-19 public health emergency when you get it from a Medicare provider or supplier.

Over-the-counter (OTC) tests:

- If you have Part B, Medicare will cover up to 8 over-the-counter COVID-19 tests at any participating pharmacy or health care provider for each calendar month until the COVID-19 public health emergency ends.
- If you're in a Medicare Advantage Plan, you won't get this benefit through your plan, but the tests will be covered directly through Part B. Check with your plan to see if it covers additional over-the-counter COVID-19 tests.
- You pay nothing for these tests during the public health emergency.
- If you have other coverage, you may be able to get free tests through that other coverage.

Get more information

- Learn more about these covered services at

Medicare.gov/medicare-coronavirus.

- For more on COVID-19, visit CDC.gov/coronavirus.

Defibrillators

Medicare may cover an implantable automatic defibrillator if you've been diagnosed with heart failure. If the surgery takes place in an outpatient setting, you pay 20% of the Medicare-approved amount for your doctors' services. You also pay a copayment. In most cases, the copayment can't be more than the Part A hospital stay deductible. The Part B deductible applies. Part A covers surgeries to implant defibrillators in an inpatient hospital setting. See inpatient hospital care on pages 27–28.

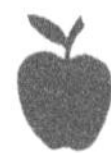

Preventive service

Depression screening

Medicare covers one depression screening per year. The screening must be done in a primary care setting (like a doctor's office) that can provide follow-up treatment and/or referrals. You pay nothing for this screening if your doctor accepts assignment.

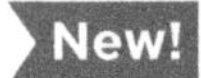

If you or someone you know is struggling or in crisis and would like to talk to a trained crisis counselor, **call or text 988**, the free and confidential Suicide & Crisis Lifeline. You can also connect with a counselor through web chat at **988lifeline.org**.

Preventive service

Diabetes screenings

Medicare covers up to 2 blood glucose (blood sugar) laboratory test screenings (with and without a carbohydrate challenge) each year if your doctor determines you're at risk for developing diabetes. You pay nothing for the test if your doctor or other qualified health care provider accepts assignment.

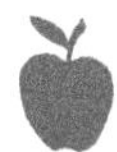

Preventive service

Diabetes self-management training

Medicare covers diabetes outpatient self-management training to teach you to cope with and manage your diabetes. The program may include tips for eating healthy, being active, monitoring blood glucose (blood sugar), taking prescription drugs, and reducing risks. You must have been diagnosed with diabetes and have a written order from your doctor or other health care provider. Some patients may also be eligible for medical nutrition therapy services (see page 46). You pay 20% of the Medicare-approved amount. The Part B deductible applies.

Diabetes equipment, supplies, & therapeutic shoes

Medicare covers meters that measure blood glucose (blood sugar) and related supplies, including test strips, lancets, lancet holders, and control solutions. Medicare also covers tubing, insertion sets, and insulin for patients using insulin pumps, and sensors for patients using continuous glucose monitors. In addition, Medicare covers one pair of extra-depth or custom shoes and inserts per year for people with specific diabetes-related foot problems.

You pay 20% of the Medicare-approved amount if your supplier accepts assignment. The Part B deductible applies.

Note: Medicare drug coverage (Part D) may cover insulin, certain medical supplies used to inject insulin (like syringes), disposable pumps, and some oral diabetes drugs. Check with your plan for more information.

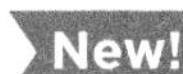

The cost of a one-month supply of insulin is capped at $35. See page 88.

Doctor & other health care provider services

Medicare covers medically necessary doctor services (including outpatient services and some inpatient hospital doctor services) and covered preventive services. Medicare also covers services you get from other health care providers, like physician assistants, nurse practitioners, clinical nurse specialists, clinical social workers, physical therapists, occupational therapists, speech-language pathologists, and clinical psychologists. Except for certain preventive services (for which you may pay nothing if your doctor or other provider accepts assignment), you pay 20% of the Medicare-approved amount for most services. The Part B deductible applies.

Important! If you haven't received services from your doctor or group practice in the last 3 years, you may be considered a new patient. Check with the doctor or group practice to see if they're accepting new patients.

Drugs

Part B covers a limited number of outpatient prescription drugs, like:

- Injections you get in a doctor's office
- Certain oral anti-cancer drugs
- Drugs used with some types of durable medical equipment (like a nebulizer or external infusion pump)
- Certain drugs you get in a hospital outpatient setting (under very limited circumstances)

For some drugs used with an external infusion pump, Medicare may also cover services (like nursing visits) under the home infusion therapy benefit (see page 44). Part B also covers some injectable or implantable drugs to treat substance use disorder when a provider administers it in a doctor's office or a hospital as an outpatient. You pay 20% of the Medicare-approved amount for these covered drugs. The Part B deductible applies. You won't have to pay any copayments for these services if you get them from a Medicare-enrolled opioid treatment program. See pages 47–48.

If the covered drugs you get in a hospital outpatient setting are part of your outpatient services, you pay a copayment for the services. However, Part B doesn't cover other types of drugs in a hospital outpatient setting (sometimes called "self-administered drugs" or drugs you'd normally take on your own). What you pay depends on whether you have Medicare drug coverage or other drug coverage, whether your drug plan covers the drug, and whether the hospital's pharmacy is in your drug plan's network. Contact your drug plan to find out what you pay for drugs you get in a hospital outpatient setting that Part B doesn't cover.

Note: Other than the examples above, you pay 100% for most drugs, unless you have Medicare drug coverage (Part D) or other drug coverage. See pages 79–90 for more information about Medicare drug coverage.

Durable medical equipment (DME)

Medicare covers medically necessary items like oxygen and oxygen equipment, wheelchairs, walkers, and hospital beds when a Medicare-enrolled doctor or other health care provider orders for use in the home. You must rent most items, but you can also buy them or some become your property after you've made a number of rental payments. You pay 20% of the Medicare-approved amount. The Part B deductible applies.

Make sure your doctors and DME suppliers are enrolled in Medicare. It's important to ask your suppliers if they participate in Medicare before you get DME. To get your DME benefits, the doctor or supplier who provides the DME must be enrolled in Medicare. If suppliers are participating suppliers, they must accept assignment (which means, they can charge you only the coinsurance and Part B deductible for the Medicare-approved amount). If DME suppliers aren't participating and don't accept assignment, there's no limit on the amount they can charge you.

Durable Medical Equipment, Prosthetics, Orthotics, & Supplies (DMEPOS) Competitive Bidding Program: If you live in or visit a competitive bidding area and need an off-the-shelf back or knee brace that's included in the DMEPOS Competitive Bidding Program, you generally must use specific suppliers called "contract suppliers," if you want Medicare to help pay for the item. Contract suppliers are required to provide the item to you and accept assignment as a term of their contract with Medicare.

To see if you live in or are visiting a competitive bidding area, or to find suppliers who accept assignment, visit

 Medicare.gov/medical-equipment-suppliers.

You can also call 1-800-MEDICARE (1-800-633-4227). TTY users can call 1-877-486-2048. You can also call 1-800-MEDICARE if you're having problems with your DME supplier, or you need to file a complaint.

Electrocardiogram (EKG or ECG) screenings

Medicare covers a routine EKG/ECG screening if you get a referral from your doctor or other health care provider during your one-time "Welcome to Medicare" visit (see page 54). After you meet the Part B deductible, you pay 20% of the Medicare-approved amount. Medicare also covers EKGs or ECGs as diagnostic tests (see page 52). You also pay a copayment if you have the test at a hospital or a hospital-owned clinic.

Emergency department services

Medicare covers these services when you have an injury, a sudden illness, or an illness that quickly gets much worse. You pay a copayment for each emergency department visit and 20% of the Medicare-approved amount for doctors' services. The Part B deductible applies. If your doctor admits you to the same hospital as an inpatient, your costs may be different.

E-visits

Medicare covers E-visits to allow you to talk with your doctor using an online patient portal without going to the doctor's office. Providers who can provide these services include doctors, nurse practitioners, clinical nurse specialists, physician assistants, physical therapists, occupational therapists, speech-language pathologists, licensed clinical social workers (in specific circumstances), and clinical psychologists (in specific circumstances).

You must talk to your doctor or other provider to start these types of services. You pay 20% of the Medicare-approved amount for your doctor's services. The Part B deductible applies.

Eyeglasses

If you have cataract surgery that implants an intraocular lens, Medicare covers one pair of eyeglasses with standard frames (or one set of contact lenses). You pay 20% of the Medicare-approved amount. The Part B deductible applies.

Note: Medicare will only pay for contact lenses or eyeglasses from a supplier enrolled in Medicare, no matter if you or your provider submits the claim.

Federally Qualified Health Center services

Federally Qualified Health Center services provide many outpatient primary care and preventive health services. There's no deductible, and you usually pay 20% of the charges or the Medicare-approved amount. You pay nothing for most preventive services. All Federally Qualified Health Centers may offer discounts if your income is limited. Visit findahealthcenter.hrsa.gov to find a health center near you.

Preventive service

Flu shots

Medicare covers the seasonal flu shot (or vaccine). You pay nothing for the flu shot if the doctor or other qualified health care provider accepts assignment for giving the shot.

Foot care

Medicare covers yearly foot exams or treatment if you have diabetes-related lower leg nerve damage that can increase the risk of limb loss or need medically necessary treatment for foot injuries or diseases, like hammer toe, bunion deformities, and heel spurs. You pay 20% of the Medicare-approved amount for medically necessary treatment your doctor approves. The Part B deductible applies. You also pay a copayment for medically necessary treatment in a hospital outpatient setting.

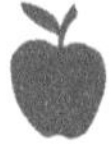

Preventive service

Glaucoma tests

Medicare covers these tests once every 12 months if you're at high risk for the eye disease glaucoma. You're at high risk if you have diabetes, a family history of glaucoma, are African American and 50 or older, or are Hispanic and 65 or older. An eye doctor who's legally allowed in your state must do or supervise the screening. You pay 20% of the Medicare-approved amount. The Part B deductible applies. You also pay a copayment in a hospital outpatient setting.

Hearing & balance exams

Medicare covers these diagnostic exams if your doctor or other health care provider orders them to see if you need medical treatment.

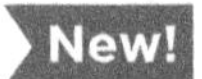

You can see an audiologist once every 12 months without an order from a doctor or other health care provider, but only for non-acute hearing conditions (like hearing loss that occurs over many years) and for diagnostic services related to hearing loss that's treated with surgically implanted hearing devices.

You pay 20% of the Medicare-approved amount. The Part B deductible applies. You also pay a copayment in a hospital outpatient setting.

Note: Medicare doesn't cover hearing aids or exams for fitting hearing aids.

Preventive service

Hepatitis B shots

Medicare covers these shots (or vaccines) if you're at medium or high risk for Hepatitis B. Some risk factors include hemophilia, End-Stage Renal Disease (ESRD), diabetes, if you live with someone who has Hepatitis B, or if you're a health care worker and have frequent contact with blood or body fluids. Check with your doctor to see if you're at medium or high risk for Hepatitis B. You pay nothing for the shot if the doctor or other qualified health care provider accepts assignment.

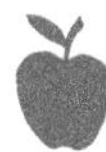

Preventive service

Hepatitis B Virus infection screenings

Medicare covers this screening if you meet one of these conditions:

- You're at high risk for Hepatitis B Virus infection.
- You're pregnant.

Medicare will only cover this screening if your primary care doctor orders it.

Medicare covers Hepatitis B Virus infection screenings:

- Yearly only if you're at continued high risk and don't get a Hepatitis B shot.
- If you're pregnant:
  - At the first prenatal visit for each pregnancy
  - At the time of delivery for those with new or continued risk factors
  - At the first prenatal visit for future pregnancies, even if you previously got the Hepatitis B shot or had negative Hepatitis B Virus screening results

You pay nothing for the screening test if the doctor or other qualified health care provider accepts assignment.

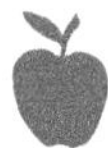

Preventive service

Hepatitis C screening tests

Medicare covers one Hepatitis C screening test if you meet one of these conditions:

- You're at high risk because you use or have used illicit injection drugs.
- You had a blood transfusion before 1992.
- You were born between 1945–1965.

Medicare also covers yearly repeat screenings if you're at high risk.

Medicare will only cover a Hepatitis C screening test if your health care provider orders one. You pay nothing for the screening test if your primary care doctor or other qualified health care provider accepts assignment.

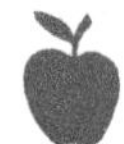

Preventive service

HIV (Human Immunodeficiency Virus) screenings

Medicare covers HIV screenings once every 12 months if you're:

- Between 15–65.
- Younger than 15 or older than 65, and at increased risk.

Medicare also covers this test up to 3 times during a pregnancy.

You pay nothing for the HIV screening if your doctor or other qualified health care provider accepts **assignment**.

Home health services

Medicare covers home health services under Part A and/or Part B. Medicare covers **medically necessary** part-time or intermittent skilled nursing care, physical therapy, speech-language pathology services, or continued occupational therapy services. Home health services may also include medical social services, part-time or intermittent home health aide services, durable medical equipment, and medical supplies for use at home. "Part-time or intermittent" means you may be able to get skilled nursing care and home health aide services if they are provided less than 8 hours each day or less than 28 hours each week (or up to 35 hours a week in some limited situations). A doctor, or other health care provider (like a nurse practitioner), must see you face-to-face before certifying that you need home health services. A doctor or other provider must order your care, and a Medicare-certified home health agency must provide it.

Medicare covers home health services as long as you need part-time or intermittent skilled services and as long as you're "homebound," which means:

- You have trouble leaving your home without help (like using a cane, wheelchair, walker, or crutches; special transportation; or help from another person) because of an illness or injury.
- Leaving your home isn't recommended because of your condition.
- You're normally unable to leave your home because it's a major effort.

You pay nothing for covered home health services. However, for Medicare-covered durable medical equipment, you pay 20% of the **Medicare-approved amount**. The Part B **deductible** applies.

Home infusion therapy services & supplies

Medicare covers equipment and supplies (like pumps, IV poles, tubing, and catheters) for home infusion therapy to administer certain IV infusion drugs at home. Certain equipment and supplies (like the infusion pump) and the infusion drug are covered under the Durable Medical Equipment benefit (see page 40). Medicare also covers services (like nursing visits), training for caregivers, and patient monitoring. You pay 20% of the Medicare-approved amount for these services and for the equipment and supplies you use in your home.

Kidney dialysis services & supplies

Generally, Medicare covers 3 dialysis treatments per week if you have End-Stage Renal Disease (ESRD). This includes most renal dialysis drugs and biological products, and all laboratory tests, home dialysis training, support services, equipment, and supplies. The dialysis facility is responsible for coordinating your dialysis services (at home or in a facility). You pay 20% of the Medicare-approved amount. The Part B deductible applies.

Kidney disease education

Medicare covers up to 6 sessions of kidney disease education services if you have Stage IV chronic kidney disease that will usually require dialysis or a kidney transplant, and your doctor or other health care provider refers you for the service. You pay 20% of the Medicare-approved amount per session if you get the service from a doctor or other qualified health care provider. The Part B deductible applies.

Laboratory tests

Medicare covers medically necessary clinical diagnostic laboratory tests when your doctor or provider orders them. These tests may include certain blood tests, urinalysis, certain tests on tissue specimens, and some screening tests. You generally pay nothing for these tests.

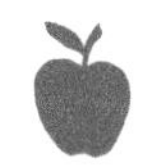

Preventive service

Lung cancer screenings

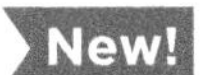

Medicare covers lung cancer screenings with low dose computed tomography once per year if you meet these updated conditions:

- You're 50–77.
- You don't have signs or symptoms of lung cancer (you're asymptomatic).
- You're either a current smoker or you quit smoking within the last 15 years.
- You have a tobacco smoking history of at least 20 "pack years" (an average of one pack—20 cigarettes—per day for 20 years).
- You get an order from your doctor.

You pay nothing for this service if your doctor accepts assignment.

Note: Before your first lung cancer screening, you'll need to schedule an appointment with your doctor to discuss the benefits and risks of lung cancer screening. You and your doctor can decide whether a lung cancer screening is right for you.

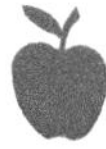

Preventive service

Mammograms

Medicare covers a mammogram screening to check for breast cancer once every 12 months if you're a woman 40 or older. Medicare covers one baseline mammogram if you're a woman between 35–39. You pay nothing for the test if the doctor or other qualified health care provider accepts assignment.

Note: Part B also covers diagnostic mammograms more frequently than once a year when medically necessary. You pay 20% of the Medicare-approved amount for diagnostic mammograms. The Part B deductible applies.

Preventive service

Medicare Diabetes Prevention Program

Medicare covers a once-per-lifetime health behavior change program to help you prevent type 2 diabetes. The program begins with weekly core sessions offered in a group setting over a 6-month period. In these sessions, you'll get:

- Training to make realistic, lasting behavior changes around diet and exercise.
- Tips on how to get more exercise.
- Strategies to control your weight.
- A specially trained coach to help keep you motivated.
- Support from people with similar goals and challenges.

Once you complete the core sessions, you'll get 6 monthly follow-up sessions to help you maintain healthy habits.

If you started the Medicare Diabetes Prevention Program in 2021 or earlier, you'll get an additional 12 monthly sessions if you meet certain weight loss goals.

To be eligible, you must have:

- Part B (or a Medicare Advantage Plan)
- A fasting plasma glucose of 110-125mg/dL, a 2-hour plasma glucose of 140-199 mg/dL (oral glucose tolerance test), or a hemoglobin A1c test result between 5.7 and 6.4% within 12 months prior to attending the first core session.
- A body mass index (BMI) of 25 or more (BMI of 23 or more if you're Asian).
- No history of type 1 or type 2 diabetes.
- You've never participated in the Medicare Diabetes Prevention Program.
- No End-Stage Renal Disease (ESRD).

You pay nothing for these services if you're eligible.

You can get them from an approved Medicare Diabetes Prevention Program supplier. These suppliers may be traditional health care providers or organizations like community centers or faith-based organizations. To find a supplier, visit Medicare.gov/talk-to-someone.

If you're in a Medicare Advantage Plan, contact your plan to find out where to get these services.

Mental health care (outpatient)

Medicare covers mental health care services to help with conditions like depression and anxiety. These visits are often called counseling or psychotherapy. Coverage includes services generally provided in an outpatient setting (like a doctor's or other health care provider's office, or hospital outpatient department), including visits with a psychiatrist or other doctor, clinical psychologist, clinical nurse specialist, clinical social worker, nurse practitioner, or physician assistant. Covered mental health care includes partial hospitalization services, which are intensive outpatient mental health services provided during the day. Partial hospitalization services are provided by a hospital to its outpatients or by a community mental health center. Visit Medicare.gov/coverage/mental-health-care-partial-hospitalization for more information.

Generally, you pay 20% of the Medicare-approved amount and the Part B deductible applies for mental health care services.

Note: Part A covers inpatient mental health care services you get in a hospital.

Preventive service

Nutrition therapy services

Medicare covers medical nutrition therapy services if you have diabetes or kidney disease, or you've had a kidney transplant in the last 36 months, and your doctor refers you for services. Only a Registered Dietitian or nutrition professional who meets certain requirements can provide medical nutrition therapy services. If you have diabetes, you may also be eligible for diabetes self-management training (see page 39). You pay nothing for medical nutrition therapy preventive services because the deductible and coinsurance don't apply.

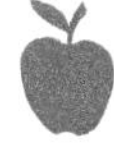

Preventive service

Obesity behavioral therapy

If you have a body mass index (BMI) of 30 or more, Medicare covers obesity screenings and behavioral counseling to help you lose weight by focusing on diet and exercise. Medicare covers this counseling if your primary care doctor or other primary care provider gives the counseling in a primary care setting (like a doctor's office), where they can coordinate your personalized prevention plan with your other care. You pay nothing for this service if the doctor or provider accepts assignment.

Occupational therapy services

Medicare covers medically necessary therapy to help you perform activities of daily living (like dressing or bathing). This therapy helps to improve or maintain current capabilities or slow decline when your doctor or other health care provider certifies you need it. You pay 20% of the Medicare-approved amount. The Part B deductible applies.

Opioid use disorder treatment services

Medicare covers opioid use disorder treatment services in opioid treatment programs. The services include medication (like methadone, buprenorphine, naltrexone, and naloxone), counseling, drug testing, individual and group therapy, intake activities, and periodic assessments. Medicare covers counseling, therapy services, and periodic assessments both in-person and, in certain circumstances, by virtual delivery (using audio and video communication technology, like your phone or a computer). Medicare also covers services given through opioid treatment program mobile units.

Medicare pays doctors and other providers for office-based opioid use disorder treatment, including management, care coordination, psychotherapy, and counseling activities.

Under Original Medicare, you won't have to pay any copayments for these services if you get them from an opioid treatment program provider that's enrolled in Medicare and meets other requirements. However, the Part B deductible still applies. Talk to your doctor or other health care provider to find out where to go for these services. You can also visit Medicare.gov/talk-to-someone to find a program near you.

Medicare Advantage Plans must also cover opioid treatment program services. If you're in a Medicare Advantage Plan, your current opioid treatment program must be Medicare-enrolled to make sure your treatment stays uninterrupted. If not, you may have to switch to a Medicare-enrolled opioid treatment program. Since Medicare Advantage Plans can apply copayments to opioid treatment program services, you should check with your plan to see if you have to pay a copayment.

Outpatient hospital services

Medicare covers many diagnostic and treatment services you get as an outpatient from a Medicare-participating hospital. Generally, you pay 20% of the Medicare-approved amount for your doctors' or other health care providers' services. You may pay more for services you get in a hospital outpatient setting than you'll pay for the same care in a doctor's office. In addition to the amount you pay the doctor, you'll also usually pay the hospital a copayment for each service you get in a hospital outpatient setting (except for certain preventive services that don't have a copayment). In most cases, the copayment can't be more than the Part A hospital stay deductible for each service. The Part B deductible applies, except for certain preventive services. If you get hospital outpatient services in a critical access hospital, your copayment may be higher and may exceed the Part A hospital stay deductible.

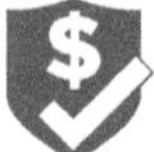

Cost & coverage: To get cost estimates for hospital outpatient procedures done in hospital outpatient departments, visit

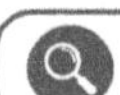 Medicare.gov/procedure-price-lookup.

Outpatient medical & surgical services & supplies

Medicare covers approved procedures, like X-rays, casts, stitches, or outpatient surgeries. You pay 20% of the Medicare-approved amount for doctor or other health care provider services. You generally pay a copayment for each service you get in a hospital outpatient setting. In most cases, the copayment can't be more than the Part A hospital stay deductible for each service you get. The Part B deductible applies, and you pay all costs for items or services that Medicare doesn't cover.

Physical therapy services

Medicare covers evaluation and treatment for injuries and diseases that change your ability to function, or to improve or maintain current function or slow decline, **when your doctor or other health care provider, including a nurse practitioner, clinical nurse specialist or physician assistant certifies you need it.** You pay 20% of the Medicare-approved amount. The Part B deductible applies.

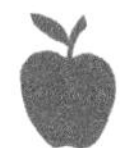

Preventive service

Pneumococcal shots

Medicare covers pneumococcal shots (or vaccines) to help prevent pneumococcal infections (like certain types of pneumonia). Medicare now covers a single dose vaccine in addition to a 2-dose series. Talk with your doctor or other health care provider to see which vaccine you should get. You pay nothing for these shots if the doctor or other qualified health care provider accepts assignment for giving the shots.

Principal care management services

Medicare covers disease-specific services to help you manage a single, complex chronic condition that puts you at risk of hospitalization, physical or cognitive decline, or death. If you have one chronic high-risk condition that you expect to last at least 3 months (like cancer and you're not being treated for any other complex conditions), Medicare may pay for a health care provider's help to manage it. Your provider will create a disease-specific care plan and continuously monitor and adjust it, including the medicines you take. The Part B deductible and coinsurance apply.

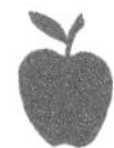

Preventive service

Prostate cancer screenings

Medicare covers digital rectal exams and prostate specific antigen (PSA) tests once every 12 months for men over 50 (starting the day after your 50th birthday). For the digital rectal exam, you pay 20% of the Medicare-approved amount. The Part B deductible applies. You also pay a copayment in a hospital outpatient setting. You pay nothing for the PSA test.

Prosthetic/orthotic items

Medicare covers these prosthetics/orthotics when a Medicare-enrolled doctor or other health care provider orders them: arm, leg, back, and neck braces; artificial eyes; artificial limbs (and their replacement parts); and prosthetic devices needed to replace an internal body organ or function of the organ (including ostomy supplies, parenteral and enteral nutrition therapy, and some types of breast prostheses after a mastectomy).

For Medicare to cover your prosthetic or orthotic, you must go to a supplier that's enrolled in Medicare. You pay 20% of the Medicare-approved amount. The Part B deductible applies.

Important! **Durable Medical Equipment, Prosthetics, Orthotics, and Supplies (DMEPOS) Competitive Bidding Program:** To get an off-the-shelf back or knee brace in most areas of the country, you generally must use specific suppliers called "contract suppliers." Otherwise, Medicare won't pay and you'll likely pay full price. See page 40.

Pulmonary rehabilitation programs

Medicare covers a comprehensive pulmonary rehabilitation program if you have:

- Moderate to very severe chronic obstructive pulmonary disease (COPD) and have a referral from your doctor to treat it.
- Had confirmed or suspected COVID-19 and experience persistent symptoms that include respiratory dysfunction for at least 4 weeks.

You pay 20% of the Medicare-approved amount if you get the service in a doctor's office. You also pay a copayment per session if you get the service in a hospital outpatient setting. The Part B deductible applies.

Rural health clinic services

Rural health clinics provide many outpatient primary care and preventive health services in rural and underserved areas. Generally, you pay 20% of the charges. The Part B deductible applies. You pay nothing for most preventive services.

Second surgical opinions

Medicare covers a second surgical opinion in some cases for medically necessary surgery that isn't an emergency. In some cases, Medicare covers third surgical opinions. You pay 20% of the Medicare-approved amount. The Part B deductible applies.

Preventive service

Sexually transmitted infection (STI) screenings & counseling

Medicare covers STI screenings for chlamydia, gonorrhea, syphilis, and/or Hepatitis B. Medicare covers these screenings if you're pregnant or at increased risk for an STI when your primary care provider orders the tests. Medicare covers these tests once every 12 months or at certain times during pregnancy.

Medicare also covers up to 2 individual, 20–30 minute, face-to-face, high-intensity behavioral counseling sessions each year if you're a sexually active adult at increased risk for STIs. Medicare will only cover these counseling sessions with a primary care doctor in a primary care setting (like a doctor's office). Medicare won't cover counseling as a preventive service in an inpatient setting, like a skilled nursing facility.

You pay nothing for these services if your primary care doctor or other qualified health care provider accepts assignment.

Shots (or vaccines)

Part B covers:

- Flu shots. See page 42.
- Hepatitis B shots. See page 43.
- Pneumococcal shots. See page 49.
- Coronavirus disease 2019 (COVID-19) vaccine. See page 37.

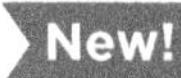
Medicare drug coverage (Part D) generally covers all other recommended adult immunizations (like shingles, tetanus, diphtheria, and pertussis vaccines) to prevent illness. **You can now get more vaccines under Part D at no cost to you.** Contact your plan for details, and talk to your provider about which ones are right for you.

Speech-language pathology services

Medicare covers medically necessary evaluation and treatment to regain and strengthen speech and language skills. This includes cognitive and swallowing skills, or to improve or maintain current function or slow decline, when your doctor or other health care provider certifies you need it. You pay 20% of the Medicare-approved amount. The Part B deductible applies.

Surgical dressing services

Medicare covers medically necessary treatment of a surgical or surgically treated wound. You pay nothing for the supplies and 20% of the Medicare-approved amount for your doctor or other health care provider services. You pay a set copayment for these services when you get them in a hospital outpatient setting. The Part B deductible applies.

Telehealth

Medicare covers certain telehealth services provided by a doctor or other heath care practitioner who's located elsewhere using audio and video communication technology (or audio-only telehealth services in some cases), like your phone or a computer. Telehealth can provide many services that generally occur in-person, including office visits, psychotherapy, consultations, and certain other medical or health services.

During the COVID-19 public health emergency and for five months after, you can get telehealth services in any location in the U.S. including your home. After this period, you must be at an office or other medical facility located in a rural area for most telehealth services.

You can get certain Medicare telehealth services **without** being in a rural health care setting, including:

- Monthly End-Stage Renal Disease (ESRD) visits for home dialysis.
- Services for diagnosis, evaluation, or treatment of symptoms of an acute stroke wherever you are, including in a mobile stroke unit.
- Services to treat a substance use disorder or a co-occurring mental health disorder (sometimes called a "dual disorder") or for the diagnosis, evaluation, or treatment of a mental health disorder in your home.

You pay 20% of the Medicare-approved amount for your doctor, other health care provider or practitioner's services. The Part B deductible applies. For most of these services, you'll pay the same amount you would if you got the services in person.

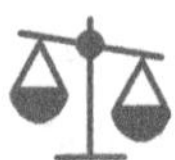

Compare: Medicare Advantage Plans and providers who are part of certain Medicare Accountable Care Organizations (ACOs) may offer more telehealth benefits than Original Medicare. For example, you may be able to get some services from home, no matter where you live. Check with your plan to see what benefits they offer. If your provider participates in an ACO, check with them to see what telehealth benefits may be available. See pages 111–112.

Tests (Non-laboratory)

Medicare covers X-rays, MRIs, CT scans, EKG/ECGs, and some other diagnostic tests. You pay 20% of the Medicare-approved amount. The Part B deductible applies.

If you get the test at a hospital as an outpatient, you also pay the hospital a copayment that may be more than 20% of the Medicare-approved amount. In most cases, this amount can't be more than the Part A hospital stay deductible. See Laboratory services on page 45 for other Part B-covered tests.

Transitional care management services

Medicare may cover this service if you're returning to your community after a stay at certain facilities, like a hospital or skilled nursing facility. The health care provider who's managing your transition back into the community will work to coordinate and manage your care for the first 30 days after you return home. They'll work with you, your family, caregivers, and other providers. You'll also get an in-person office visit within 2 weeks of your return home. The health care provider may also review information on the care you got in the facility, provide information to help you transition back to living at home, work with other care providers, help you with referrals or arrangements for follow-up care or community resources, help you with scheduling, and help you manage your medications. The Part B deductible and coinsurance apply.

Transplants & immunosuppressive drugs

Medicare covers doctor services for heart, lung, kidney, pancreas, intestine, and liver transplants under certain conditions, but only in Medicare-certified facilities. Medicare also covers bone marrow and cornea transplants under certain conditions.

Note: Medicare may cover transplant surgery as a hospital inpatient service under Part A. See pages 27–28.

Medicare covers immunosuppressive drugs if Medicare paid for the transplant. You must have Part A at the time of the covered transplant, and you must have Part B at the time you get immunosuppressive drugs. You pay 20% of the Medicare-approved amount for the drugs. The Part B deductible applies. Keep in mind, Medicare drug coverage (Part D) covers immunosuppressive drugs if Part B doesn't cover them.

If you're thinking about joining a Medicare Advantage Plan and are on a transplant waiting list or think you need a transplant, check with the plan before you join to make sure your doctors, other health care providers, and hospitals are in the plan's network. Also, check the plan's coverage rules for prior authorization.

Medicare pays the full cost of care for your kidney donor. You and your donor won't have to pay a deductible, coinsurance, or any other costs for their hospital stay.

New! **Immunosuppressive drug benefit**
If you only have Medicare because of End Stage Renal Disease (ESRD), your Medicare coverage, including immunosuppressive drug coverage, ends 36 months after a successful kidney transplant. Medicare offers a benefit that helps you pay for your immunosuppressive drugs **if you don't have certain types of other health coverage** (like a group health plan, TRICARE, or Medicaid that covers immunosuppressive drugs). **This new benefit only covers your immunosuppressive drugs and no other items or services. It isn't a substitute for full health coverage. You can sign up for this benefit anytime as long as you had Medicare because of ESRD at the time of your kidney transplant.** To sign up, call Social Security at 1-800-772-1213. TTY users can call 1-800-325-0788.

Note: You'll pay a monthly premium of $97.10* and $226 deductible for this benefit in 2023. Once you've met the deductible, you'll pay 20% of the Medicare-approved amount for immunosuppressive drugs. If you have limited income and resources, you may be able to get help from your state to pay for this benefit. See page 94, or visit Medicare.gov/basics/end-stage-renal-disease to learn more.

* You may pay a higher premium based on your income.

Travel

Medicare generally doesn't cover health care while you're traveling outside the U.S. (the "U.S." includes the 50 states, the District of Columbia, Puerto Rico, the U.S. Virgin Islands, Guam, the Northern Mariana Islands, and American Samoa). There are some exceptions, including cases where Medicare may pay for services you get while on board a ship within the territorial waters adjoining the land areas of the U.S. Medicare may pay for inpatient hospital, doctor, or ambulance services you get in a foreign country in these rare cases:

- You're in the U.S. when an emergency occurs, and the foreign hospital is closer than the nearest U.S. hospital that can treat your medical condition.
- You're traveling through Canada without unreasonable delay by the most direct route between Alaska and another U.S. state when a medical emergency occurs, and the Canadian hospital is closer than the nearest U.S. hospital that can treat the emergency.
- You live in the U.S. and the foreign hospital is closer to your home than the nearest U.S. hospital that can treat your medical condition, regardless of whether an emergency exists.

Medicare may cover medically necessary ambulance transportation to a foreign hospital only with admission for medically necessary covered inpatient hospital services. You pay 20% of the Medicare-approved amount. The Part B deductible applies.

Urgently needed care

Medicare covers urgently needed care to treat a sudden illness or injury that isn't a medical emergency. You pay 20% of the Medicare-approved amount for your doctor or other health care provider services, and a copayment in a hospital outpatient setting. The Part B deductible applies.

Virtual check-ins

Medicare covers virtual check-ins (also called "brief communication technology-based services") with your doctor or certain other providers, like nurse practitioners, clinical nurse specialists, or physician assistants, using audio and video communication technology, like your phone or a computer, without going to the doctor's office. Your doctor can also conduct remote assessments using photo or video images you send for review to see whether you need to go to the doctor's office.

Your doctor or other provider can respond to you by phone, virtual delivery, secure text message, email, or patient portal.

You can use these services if you have met these conditions:

- You talked to your doctor or other provider about starting these types of visits.
- The virtual check-in doesn't relate to a medical visit you've had within the past 7 days and doesn't lead to the medical visit within the next 24 hours (or the soonest appointment available).
- You verbally consent to the virtual check-in, and your doctor documents your consent in your medical record. Your doctor may get one consent for a year's worth of these services.

You pay 20% of the **Medicare-approved amount** for your doctor or other health care provider services. The Part B **deductible** applies.

Preventive service

"Welcome to Medicare" preventive visit

During the first 12 months that you have Part B, you can get a "Welcome to Medicare" preventive visit. The visit includes a review of your medical and social history related to your health. It also includes education and counseling about **preventive services**, including certain screenings, shots or vaccines (like flu, pneumococcal, and other recommended shots or vaccines), and **referrals** for other care, if needed.

When you make your appointment, let your doctor's office know that you'd like to schedule your "Welcome to Medicare" preventive visit. You pay nothing for the "Welcome to Medicare" preventive visit if the doctor or other qualified health care provider accepts **assignment**.

If you have a current prescription for opioids, your provider will review your potential risk factors for opioid use disorder, evaluate your severity of pain and current treatment plan, provide information on non-opioid treatment options, and may refer you to a specialist, if appropriate. Your provider will also review your potential risk factors for substance use disorder, like **alcohol and tobacco use**, and refer you for treatment, if needed.

Important! If your doctor or other health care provider performs additional tests or services during the same visit that Medicare doesn't cover under this preventive benefit, you may have to pay **coinsurance**, and the Part B deductible may apply. If Medicare doesn't cover the additional tests or services (like a routine physical exam), you may have to pay the full amount.

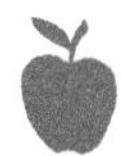

Preventive service

Yearly "Wellness" visit

If you've had Part B for longer than 12 months, you can get a yearly "Wellness" visit to develop or update your personalized plan to prevent disease or disability based on your current health and risk factors. **The yearly "Wellness" visit isn't a physical exam.** Medicare covers this visit once every 12 months.

Your provider will ask you to fill out a questionnaire, called a "Health Risk Assessment," as part of this visit. Answering these questions can help you and your provider develop a personalized prevention plan to help you stay healthy and get the most out of your visit. Your visit may include: routine measurements, health advice, a review of your medical and family history, your current prescriptions, advance care planning and more.

Your provider will also perform a cognitive assessment to look for signs of dementia, including Alzheimer's disease. Signs of cognitive impairment include trouble remembering, learning new things, concentrating, managing finances, and making decisions about your everyday life. If your provider thinks you may have cognitive impairment, Medicare covers a separate visit to do a more thorough review of your cognitive function and check for conditions like dementia, depression, anxiety, or delirium and design a care plan. See pages 34–35.

Your provider will also evaluate your potential risk factors for a substance use disorder and refer you for treatment, if needed. If you use opioid medication, your provider will review your pain treatment plan, share information about non-opioid treatment options, and refer you to a specialist, as appropriate.

Note: Your first yearly "Wellness" visit can't take place within 12 months of your Part B enrollment or your "Welcome to Medicare" preventive visit. However, you don't need to have had a "Welcome to Medicare" preventive visit to qualify for a yearly "Wellness" visit.

You pay nothing for the yearly "Wellness" visit if the doctor or other qualified health care provider accepts assignment.

Important! If your doctor or other health care provider performs additional tests or services during the same visit that Medicare doesn't cover under this preventive benefit, you may have to pay a coinsurance, and the Part B deductible may apply. If Medicare doesn't cover the additional tests or services (like a routine physical exam), you may have to pay the full amount.

What's NOT covered by Part A and Part B?

Medicare doesn't cover everything. If you need certain services Part A or Part B doesn't cover, you'll have to pay for them yourself unless:

- You have other coverage (including Medicaid) to cover the costs.
- You're in a Medicare Advantage Plan or Medicare Cost Plan that covers these services. Medicare Advantage Plans and Medicare Cost Plans may cover some extra benefits, like fitness programs and vision, hearing, and dental services.

Some of the items and services that Original Medicare doesn't cover include:

- ✖ Most dental care*
- ✖ Eye exams (for prescription glasses)
- ✖ Dentures
- ✖ Long-term care
- ✖ Cosmetic surgery
- ✖ Massage therapy
- ✖ Routine physical exams
- ✖ Hearing aids and exams for fitting them
- ✖ Concierge care (also called concierge medicine, retainer-based medicine, boutique medicine, platinum practice, or direct care)
- ✖ Covered items or services you get from an opt-out doctor (see page 60) or other provider (except in the case of an emergency or urgent need)

* **Note:** Original Medicare may pay for some dental services before, or as part of, certain related medical procedures (like before certain cardiac or organ transplant procedures).

Paying for long-term care

Medicare and most health insurance, including Medicare Supplement Insurance (Medigap), don't pay for long-term care. This type of care (sometimes called "long-term services and supports") includes medical and non-medical care for people who have a chronic illness or disability. This includes personal care assistance, like help with everyday activities, including dressing, bathing and using the bathroom. Long-term care may also include home-delivered meals, adult day health care, and other services. You may be eligible for this care through Medicaid, or you can choose to buy private long-term care insurance.

You can get long-term care at home, in the community, in an assisted living facility, or in a nursing home. It's important to start planning for long-term care now to maintain your independence and to make sure you get the care you may need, in the setting you want, now and in the future.

Long-term care resources

Use these resources to get more information about long-term care:

- Visit longtermcare.acl.gov to learn more about planning for long-term care.
- Call your State Insurance Department to get information about long-term care insurance. Call 1-800-MEDICARE (1-800-633-4227) to get the phone number. TTY users can call 1-877-486-2048.
- Call your State Medical Assistance (Medicaid) office or visit Medicaid.gov and ask for information about long-term care coverage.
- Get a copy of "A Shopper's Guide to Long-Term Care Insurance" from the National Association of Insurance Commissioners at content.naic.org/sites/default/files/publication-ltc-lp-shoppers-guide-long-term.pdf.
- Call your State Health Insurance Assistance Program (SHIP). See pages 115–118 for the phone number of your local SHIP.
- Visit the Eldercare Locator at eldercare.acl.gov to find help in your community.

SECTION 3

Original Medicare

How does Original Medicare work?

Original Medicare is one of your Medicare health coverage choices. You'll have Original Medicare unless you choose a **Medicare Advantage Plan** or other type of **Medicare health plan**.

You generally have to pay a portion of the cost for each service Original Medicare covers. There's no limit to what you'll pay out of pocket in a year unless you have other coverage (like **Medigap**, **Medicaid**, or employee or union coverage) or join a Medicare Advantage Plan. See page 59 for the general rules about how your costs work.

Original Medicare

Can I get my health care from any doctor, other health care provider, or hospital?	In most cases, yes. You can go to any Medicare-enrolled doctor, other health care provider, hospital, or other facility that accepts Medicare patients anywhere in the U.S. Visit **Medicare.gov/care-compare** to find and compare providers, hospitals, and facilities in your area.
Does it cover prescription drugs?	No, with a few exceptions (see pages 26–27, 47, and 51), Original Medicare doesn't cover most drugs. You can add Medicare drug coverage (Part D) by joining a separate Medicare drug plan. See pages 79–90.
Do I need to choose a primary care doctor?	No.
Do I have to get a referral to see a specialist?	In most cases, no.
Should I get a supplemental policy?	You may already have Medicaid, military retiree, or employer or union coverage that may pay costs that Original Medicare doesn't. If not, you may want to buy a Medicare Supplement Insurance (Medigap) policy if you're eligible. See pages 75–78.

Note: See pages 119–122 for definitions of **blue** words.

What else do I need to know about Original Medicare?	• You generally pay a set amount for your health care (deductible) before Medicare begins to pay its share. Once Medicare pays its share, you pay a coinsurance or copayment for covered services and supplies. **There's no yearly limit for what you pay out of pocket** unless you have other insurance (like Medigap, Medicaid, or employee, retiree, or union coverage). • You usually pay a monthly premium for Part B. • You generally don't need to file Medicare claims. Providers and suppliers must file your claims for the covered services and supplies you get.

What do I pay?

Your out-of-pocket costs in Original Medicare depend on:

- Whether you have Part A and/or Part B. Most people have both.
- Whether your doctor, other health care provider, or supplier accepts "assignment." See page 59.
- The type of health care you need and how often you need it.
- If you choose to get services or supplies Medicare doesn't cover. If so, you pay all costs unless you have other insurance that covers them.
- Whether you have other health insurance that works with Medicare.
- Whether you have full Medicaid or get help from your state to pay your Medicare costs through a Medicare Savings Program. See pages 94–95.
- Whether you have Medicare Supplement Insurance (Medigap).
- Whether you and your doctor or other health care provider sign a private contract. See page 60.

How do I know what Medicare paid?

If you have Original Medicare, you'll get a "Medicare Summary Notice" (MSN) that lists all the services billed to Medicare. You can sign up to get this Notice electronically every month (see below) or a Medicare contractor will mail it to you every 3 months. It's not a bill. The MSN shows what Medicare paid and what you may owe the provider. Review your MSNs to be sure you got all the services, supplies, or equipment listed. If you disagree with Medicare's decision not to pay for (cover) a service, the MSN will tell you how to appeal. See page 99 for information on how to file an appeal.

If you need to change your address on your MSN, call Social Security at 1-800-772-1213. TTY users can call 1-800-325-0778. If you get Railroad Retirement Board (RRB) benefits, call the RRB at 1-877-772-5772. TTY users can call 1-312-751-4701.

Your MSN will tell you if you're enrolled in the Qualified Medicare Beneficiary (QMB) program. If you're in the QMB program, Medicare providers aren't allowed to bill you for Medicare Part A and/or Part B deductibles, coinsurance, or copayments. In some cases, you may be billed a small copayment through Medicaid, if one applies. For more information about QMB and steps to take if a provider bills you for these costs, see page 94.

Important! **Get your Medicare Summary Notices electronically**

Sign up to get your "Medicare Summary Notices," (also called "eMSNs") electronically. Visit Medicare.gov to log into (or create) your secure Medicare account. If you sign up for eMSNs, we'll send you an email each month when they're available in your Medicare account. The eMSNs have the same information as paper MSNs. You won't get printed copies in the mail if you choose eMSNs. As of 2021, people who signed up for eMSNs helped save the Medicare Program close to $18 million.

You have options in how you get your Medicare claims information. A growing number of computer and mobile apps are connected to Medicare through Blue Button 2.0. If you agree to share your information with one of these apps, it can show you the details of the claims that Medicare has paid on your behalf. See pages 109–110 for more information.

What's assignment?

Assignment means that your doctor, provider, or supplier agrees (or is required by law) to accept the Medicare-approved amount as full payment for covered services.

If your doctor, provider, or supplier accepts assignment:

- Your out-of-pocket costs may be less.
- They agree to charge you only the Medicare deductible and coinsurance amount and usually wait for Medicare to pay its share before asking you to pay your share.
- They have to submit your claim directly to Medicare and can't charge you for submitting the claim.

Some providers haven't agreed and aren't required by law to accept assignment for all Medicare-covered services, but they can still choose to accept assignment for individual services. The providers who haven't agreed to accept assignment for all services are called "non-participating." You might have to pay more for their services if they don't accept assignment for the care they provide to you. Here's what happens if your doctor, provider, or supplier doesn't accept assignment:

- **You might have to pay the entire charge at the time of service.** Your doctor, provider, or supplier is supposed to submit a claim to Medicare for any Medicare-covered services they provide to you. If they don't submit the Medicare claim once you ask them to, call 1-800-MEDICARE (1-800-633-4227). TTY users can call 1-877-486-2048.
- **They can charge you more than the Medicare-approved amount. In many cases, the charge can't be more than an amount called "the limiting charge."**

If you have Original Medicare, you can see any provider you want that takes Medicare, anywhere in the U.S.

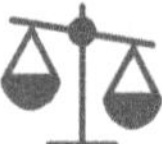

Compare: If you're in a Medicare Advantage Plan, in most cases, you'll need to use doctors and other providers who are in the plan's network.

To find out if someone accepts assignment or participates in Medicare, visit

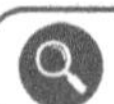 Medicare.gov/care-compare.

To find out if a medical equipment supplier accepts assignment, visit

 Medicare.gov/medical-equipment-suppliers.

You can also contact your State Health Insurance Assistance Program (SHIP) to get free help with these topics. See pages 115–118 for the phone number of your local SHIP.

What if I want to use a provider who opts out of Medicare?

Certain doctors and other health care providers who don't want to work with the Medicare Program may "opt out" of Medicare. Medicare doesn't pay for any covered items or services you get from an opt-out doctor or other provider, except in the case of an emergency or urgent need. If you still want to see an opt-out provider, you and your provider can set up payment terms that you both agree to through a private contract.

A doctor or other provider who chooses to opt out must do so for 2 years, which automatically renews every 2 years unless the provider requests not to renew their opt-out status. You can still get care from these providers, but they must enter into a private contract with you (unless you're in need of emergency or urgently needed care).

If you're unsure if a provider has opted out of Medicare, check with them so you'll know ahead of time if you'll need to pay out-of-pocket for your care.

SECTION 4

Medicare Advantage Plans & other options

What are Medicare Advantage Plans?

A Medicare Advantage Plan is another way to get your Medicare Part A and Part B coverage. Medicare Advantage Plans, sometimes called "Part C" or "MA Plans," are offered by Medicare-approved private companies that must follow rules set by Medicare. Most Medicare Advantage Plans include drug coverage (Part D). In most cases, you'll need to use health care providers who participate in the plan's network. These plans set a limit on what you'll have to pay out-of-pocket each year for covered services. Some plans offer non-emergency coverage out of network, but typically at a higher cost. In many cases, you may need to get approval from your plan before it covers certain drugs or services.

Remember, you must use the card from your Medicare Advantage Plan to get your Medicare-covered services. Keep your red, white, and blue Medicare card in a safe place because you might need it later.

If you join a Medicare Advantage Plan, you'll still have Medicare but you'll get most of your Part A and Part B coverage from your Medicare Advantage Plan, not Original Medicare.

What are the different types of Medicare Advantage Plans?

- **Health Maintenance Organization (HMO) plan:** See page 66.
- **HMO Point-of-Service (HMOPOS) plan:** This HMO plan may allow you to get some services out of network for a higher copayment or coinsurance. See page 66.
- **Medical Savings Account (MSA) plans:** See page 67.
- **Preferred Provider Organization (PPO) plan:** See page 68.
- **Private Fee-for-Service (PFFS) plan:** See page 69.
- **Special Needs Plan (SNP):** See page 70.

What do Medicare Advantage Plans cover?

Medicare Advantage Plans provide all of your Part A and Part B benefits, excluding clinical trials (clinical research studies), hospice services, and, for a temporary time, some new benefits that come from legislation or national coverage determinations. Be sure to contact your plan if you have questions about covered services.

Note: See pages 119–122 for definitions of blue words.

Plans may offer some extra benefits
With a Medicare Advantage Plan, you may have coverage for things Original Medicare doesn't cover, like fitness programs (gym memberships or discounts) and some vision, hearing, and dental services (like routine check ups or cleanings). Plans can also choose to cover even more benefits. For example, some plans may offer coverage for services like transportation to doctor visits, over-the-counter drugs that Part D doesn't cover, and services that promote your health and wellness. Check with the plan before you join to see what benefits it offers, and if there are any limitations.

Plans can also tailor their benefit packages to offer additional benefits to certain chronically-ill enrollees. These packages will provide benefits customized to treat specific conditions. Although you can check with a Medicare Advantage plan before you join to see if they offer these benefit packages, you'll need to wait until you join the plan to see if you qualify.

Get the most out of your dental benefits
If you're in a Medicare Advantage Plan, take charge of your oral health, and contact your plan to learn more about dental services that may be covered and what limitations may apply.

Medicare Advantage Plans must follow Medicare's rules

Medicare pays a fixed amount for your coverage each month to the companies offering Medicare Advantage Plans. These companies must follow rules set by Medicare. However, each Medicare Advantage Plan can charge different out-of-pocket costs and have different rules for how you get services (like whether you need a referral to see a specialist or if you have to go to doctors, facilities, or suppliers that belong to the plan's network for non-emergency or non-urgent care). These rules can change each year. The plan must notify you about any changes before the start of the next enrollment year.

Remember, you have the option each year to keep your current plan, choose a different plan, or switch to Original Medicare. See page 71.

Providers can join or leave a plan's provider network any time during the year. Your plan can also change the providers in the network any time during the year. If this happens, you usually won't be able to change plans but you can choose a new provider. You generally can't change plans during the year.

Even though the network of providers may change during the year, the plan must still give you access to qualified doctors and specialists. Your plan should make a good faith effort to give you at least 30 days' notice that your provider is leaving your plan so you have time to choose a new provider. You'll get this notice if you see that provider regularly or if it's your primary care provider. Your plan should also help you choose a new provider to continue managing your health care needs, and will help you continue needed care that's already in progress. Read your notices carefully so you're aware of any changes and can change plans if you aren't satisfied.

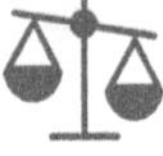

Compare: In most cases, you don't need a referral to see a specialist if you have Original Medicare (see page 57). You can also see any provider you want that takes Medicare, anywhere in the U.S.

Important!

Read the information you get from your plan

If you're in a Medicare Advantage Plan, review the "Annual Notice of Change" and "Evidence of Coverage" (EOC) from your plan each year:

- **Annual Notice of Change:** Includes any changes in coverage, costs, and more that will be effective starting in January. Your plan will send you a printed copy by September 30.
- **Evidence of Coverage:** Gives you details about what the plan covers, how much you pay, and more in the next year. Your plan will send you a notice (or printed copy) by October 15, which will include information on how to access the Evidence of Coverage electronically or request a printed copy.

If you decide to join a Medicare Advantage Plan, consider signing up for an electronic version of the Medicare & You handbook. You'll get cost and coverage information from your plan. If you don't get these important documents, contact your plan.

What should I know about Medicare Advantage Plans?

Who can join?

To join a Medicare Advantage Plan you must:

- Have Part A and Part B.
- Live in the plan's service area.
- Be a U.S. citizen or lawfully present in the U.S.

Joining and leaving

- You can join a Medicare Advantage Plan even if you have a pre-existing condition.
- **You can join or drop a Medicare Advantage Plan only at certain times during the year.** See pages 71–72.
- Each year, Medicare Advantage Plans can choose to leave Medicare or make changes in coverage, costs, service area, and more. If the plan decides to stop participating in Medicare, you'll have to join another Medicare Advantage Plan or return to Original Medicare. See page 98.
- Medicare Advantage Plans must follow certain rules when giving you information about how to join their plan. See pages 105–106 for more information about these rules and how to protect your personal information.

What if I have End-Stage Renal Disease (ESRD)?

If you have ESRD, you can choose either Original Medicare or a Medicare Advantage Plan when deciding how to get Medicare coverage. You can join a Medicare Advantage Plan during Open Enrollment (October 15–December 7, 2022). Your plan coverage starts January 1, 2023. If you're only eligible for Medicare because you have ESRD and you get a kidney transplant, your Medicare benefits will end 36 months after the transplant. See page 52 for more information.

Medicare drug coverage (Part D)
Most Medicare Advantage Plans include Medicare drug coverage (Part D). In certain types of plans that don't include Medicare drug coverage (like Medical Savings Account Plans and some Private-Fee-for-Service Plans), you can join a separate Medicare drug plan. However, if you join a Health Maintenance Organization or Preferred Provider Organization Plan which doesn't cover drugs, you can't join a separate Medicare drug plan.

In this case, you'll either need to use other prescription drug coverage you have (like employer or retiree coverage), or go without drug coverage. If you decide not to get Medicare drug coverage when you're first eligible and your other drug coverage isn't creditable prescription drug coverage, you may have to pay a late enrollment penalty if you join a plan later.

What if I have other coverage?
Talk to your employer, union, or other benefits administrator about their rules before you join a Medicare Advantage Plan. In some cases, joining a Medicare Advantage Plan might cause you to lose your employer or union coverage for yourself, your spouse, and your dependents, and you may not be able to get it back. In other cases, if you join a Medicare Advantage Plan, you may still be able to use your employer or union coverage along with the Medicare Advantage Plan you join. Your employer or union may also offer a Medicare Advantage retiree health plan that they sponsor. You can only be in one Medicare Advantage Plan at a time.

What if I have Medicare Supplement Insurance (Medigap)?
You can't buy (and can't use) Medigap while you're in a Medicare Advantage Plan. You can't use Medigap to pay for any costs (copayments, deductibles, and premiums) you have with a Medicare Advantage Plan.

Important! If you already have Medigap and join a Medicare Advantage Plan, you may want to drop Medigap. **Keep in mind, if you drop Medigap to join a Medicare Advantage Plan, you may not be able to get it back depending on your state's Medigap enrollment rules and your situation.** See page 78.

What do I pay?
Your out-of-pocket costs in a Medicare Advantage Plan depend on:

- Whether the plan charges a monthly premium. Some Medicare Advantage Plans have a $0 premium (but you still may pay the Part B premium). If you join a plan that does charge a premium, you pay this in addition to the Part B premium (and the Part A premium if you don't have premium-free Part A).
- Whether the plan pays any of your monthly Part B premiums. Some Medicare Advantage Plans will help pay all or part of your Part B premium. This is sometimes called a "Medicare Part B premium reduction."
- Whether the plan has a yearly deductible or any additional deductibles for certain services.
- How much you pay for each visit or service (copayments or coinsurance). Medicare Advantage Plans can't charge more than Original Medicare for certain services, like chemotherapy, dialysis, and skilled nursing facility care.
- The type of health care services you need and how often you get them.

- Whether you get services from a network provider or a provider that doesn't contract with the plan. If you go to a doctor, other health care provider, facility, or supplier that doesn't belong to the plan's network for non-emergency or non-urgent care services, your plan may not cover your services, or your costs could be higher.
- Whether you go to a doctor or supplier who accepts assignment (if you're in a Preferred Provider Organization or Private Fee-for-Service plan, or Medical Savings Account plan and you go out of network). See page 59 for more information about assignment.
- Whether the plan offers extra benefits (in addition to Original Medicare benefits) and if you need to pay extra to get them.
- The plan's yearly limit on your out-of-pocket costs for all Part A and Part B medical services. Once you reach this limit, you'll pay nothing for Part A- and Part B-covered services.
- Whether you have Medicaid or get help from your state through a Medicare Savings Program. See pages 94–95.

To learn more about your costs in a specific Medicare Advantage Plan, contact the plan or visit Medicare.gov/plan-compare.

How do I find out if my plan covers a service, drug, or supply?
You or your provider can get a decision, either orally or in writing, from your plan in advance to see if it covers a service, drug, or supply. You can also find out how much you'll have to pay. **This is called an "organization determination."** Sometimes you have to do this as prior authorization for your plan to cover the service, drug, or supply.

You, your representative, or your doctor can request an organization determination. The requested organization determination can be either oral or written. Based on your health needs, you, your representative, or your doctor can ask for a fast decision on your organization determination request. If your plan denies coverage, the plan must tell you in writing, and you have the right to appeal. See pages 97–101.

If a plan provider refers you for a covered service or to a provider outside the network, but doesn't get an organization determination in advance, **this is called "plan directed care."** In most cases, you won't have to pay more than the plan's usual cost sharing. Check with your plan for more information about this protection.

Types of Medicare Advantage Plans

HMO Health Maintenance Organization (HMO) plan

Can I get my health care from any doctor, other health care provider, or hospital?
No. You generally must get your care and services from doctors, other health care providers, or hospitals in the plan's network (except for emergency care, out-of-area urgent care, or temporary out-of-area dialysis, which is covered whether it's provided in the plan's network or outside the plan's network). However, some HMO plans, known as HMO Point-of-Service (HMOPOS) plans, offer an out-of-network benefit for some or all covered benefits.

Do these plans cover prescription drugs?
In most cases, yes. If you're planning to enroll in an HMO and you want Medicare drug coverage (Part D), you must join an HMO plan that offers Medicare drug coverage. If you join an HMO plan without drug coverage, you can't join a separate Medicare drug plan.

Do I need to choose a primary care doctor?
In most cases, yes.

Do I have to get a referral to see a specialist?
In most cases, yes. Certain services, like yearly screening mammograms, don't require a referral.

What else do I need to know about this type of plan?
- If you get non-emergency health care outside the plan's network without authorization, you may have to pay the full cost.
- It's important that you follow the plan's rules, like getting prior approval for a certain service when needed.
- Check with the plan for more information.

Note: HMOPOS plans (a type of HMO plan) may allow you to get some services out of network for a higher copayment or coinsurance.

MSA

Medical Savings Account (MSA) plan

Can I get my health care from any doctor, other health care provider, or hospital?
Yes. MSA plans usually don't have a network of doctors, other health care providers, or hospitals.

Do these plans cover prescription drugs?
No. If you join a Medicare MSA plan and want Medicare drug coverage (Part D), you'll have to join a separate Medicare drug plan.

Do I need to choose a primary care doctor?
No.

Do I have to get a referral to see a specialist?
No.

What else do I need to know about this type of plan?
The plan deposits money into a special savings account for you to use to pay health care expenses. The amount of the deposit varies by plan. You can use this money to pay your Medicare-covered costs before you meet the deductible. Money left in your account at the end of the year stays there. If you keep your plan the following year, your plan will add any new deposits to the amount left over.

- MSA plans don't charge a premium, but you must continue to pay your Part B premium.
- The plan will only begin to cover your costs once you meet a high yearly deductible, which varies by plan.
- Some plans may cover some extra benefits, like vision, hearing, and dental services. You may pay a premium for this extra coverage.
- For more information about using your MSA plan, visit Medicare.gov or check with your plan.

PPO Preferred Provider Organization (PPO) plan

Can I get my health care from any doctor, other health care provider, or hospital?
Yes. PPO plans have network doctors, specialists, hospitals, and other health care providers you can use. You can also use out-of-network providers for covered services, usually for a higher cost, if the provider agrees to treat you and hasn't opted out of Medicare (for Medicare Part A and Part B items and services). You're always covered for emergency and urgent care.

Do these plans cover prescription drugs?
In most cases, yes. If you're planning to enroll in a PPO and you want Medicare drug coverage (Part D), you must join a PPO plan that offers Medicare drug coverage. If you join a PPO plan without drug coverage, you can't join a separate Medicare drug plan.

Do I need to choose a primary care doctor?
No.

Do I have to get a referral to see a specialist?
In most cases, no. But if you use plan specialists (in network), your costs for covered services will usually be lower than if you use non-plan specialists (out of network).

What else do I need to know about this type of plan?
- Because certain providers are "preferred," you can save money by using them.
- Check with the plan for more information.

PFFS

Private Fee-for-Service (PFFS) plan

Can I get my health care from any doctor, other health care provider, or hospital?
You can go to any Medicare-approved doctor, other health care provider, or hospital that accepts the plan's payment terms, agrees to treat you, and hasn't opted out of Medicare (for Medicare Part A and Part B items and services). If you join a PFFS plan that has a network, you can also see any of the network providers who have agreed to always treat plan members. If you choose an out-of-network doctor, hospital, or other provider who accepts the plan's terms, you may pay more.

Do these plans cover prescription drugs?
Sometimes. If your PFFS plan doesn't offer Medicare drug coverage, you can join a separate Medicare drug plan to get Medicare drug coverage (Part D).

Do I need to choose a primary care doctor?
No.

Do I have to get a referral to see a specialist?
No.

What else do I need to know about this type of plan?

- The plan decides how much you pay for services. The plan will tell you about your cost sharing in the "Annual Notice of Change" and "Evidence of Coverage" documents that it sends each year.
- Some PFFS plans contract with a network of providers who agree to always treat you, even if you've never seen them before.
- Out-of-network doctors, hospitals, and other providers may decide not to treat you, even if you've seen them before.
- In a medical emergency, doctors, hospitals, and other providers must treat you.
- For each service you get, make sure to show your plan member card before you get treated.
- Check with the plan for more information.

SNP

Special Needs Plan (SNP)

A SNP provides benefits and services to people with specific diseases, certain health care needs, or who also have Medicaid coverage. SNPs tailor their benefits, provider choices, and list of drugs (formularies) to best meet the specific needs of the groups they serve.

Can I get my health care from any doctor, other health care provider, or hospital?
Some SNPs cover services out of network and some don't. Check with the plan to see if they cover services out of network, and if so, how it affects your costs.

Do these plans cover prescription drugs?
Yes. All SNPs must provide Medicare drug coverage (Part D).

Do I need to choose a primary care doctor?
Some SNPs require primary care doctors and some don't. Check with the plan to see if you need to choose a primary care doctor.

Do I have to get a referral to see a specialist?
Some SNPs require referrals and some don't. Certain services, like yearly screening mammograms, don't require a referral. Check with the plan to see if you need a referral.

What else do I need to know about this type of plan?

- These groups are eligible to enroll in a SNP:
  - People who live in certain institutions (like nursing homes) or who live in the community but require nursing care at home (also called an "Institutional SNP" or I-SNP).
  - People who are eligible for both Medicare and Medicaid (also called a "Dual Eligible SNP" or D-SNP). D-SNPs contract with your state Medicaid program to help coordinate your Medicare and Medicaid benefits.
  - People who have specific severe or disabling chronic conditions (like diabetes, End-Stage Renal Disease (ESRD), HIV/AIDS, chronic heart failure, or dementia) (also called a "Chronic condition SNP" or C-SNP). Plans may further limit membership to a single chronic condition or a group of related chronic conditions.
- A SNP provides benefits targeted to its members' special needs, including care coordination services.
- To find and compare Medicare Advantage Plans, visit:

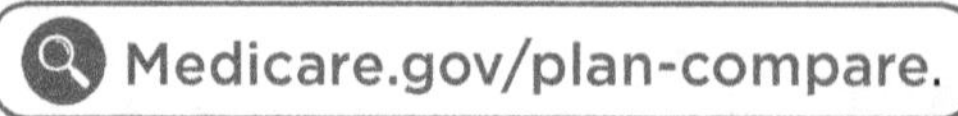

Select "Special Needs Plans" to see if a SNP is available in your area. If you need more information, check with the plan.

You can join, switch, drop, or make changes to your Medicare Advantage Plan

Initial Enrollment Period See page 17.	**When you first become eligible for Medicare**	When you first become eligible for Medicare, you can join a Medicare Advantage Plan. If you joined a Medicare Advantage Plan during your Initial Enrollment Period, you can switch to another Medicare Advantage Plan (with or without drug coverage) or go back to Original Medicare (with or without a separate Medicare drug plan) within the first 3 months you have Medicare.
General Enrollment Period See page 18.	**January 1 to March 31**	If you have Part A coverage and you get Part B for the first time during this period, you can also join a Medicare Advantage Plan. **New!** Your coverage starts the first day of the month after you sign up. Remember, you must have both Part A and Part B to join a Medicare Advantage Plan.
Open Enrollment Period	**October 15 to December 7**	You can join, switch, or drop a Medicare Advantage Plan during the Open Enrollment Period each year. Your coverage starts on January 1 (as long as the plan gets your request by December 7). If you join a Medicare Advantage Plan during this period but change your mind, you can switch back to Original Medicare or change to a different Medicare Advantage Plan (depending on which coverage works better for you) during the Medicare Advantage Open Enrollment Period (January 1 – March 31).

<table>
<tr><td>Medicare Advantage Open Enrollment Period</td><td>January 1 to March 31

Note: You can only switch plans once during this period.</td><td>If you're in a Medicare Advantage Plan (with or without drug coverage), during this period you can:<ul><li>Switch to another Medicare Advantage Plan (with or without drug coverage).</li><li>Drop your Medicare Advantage Plan and return to Original Medicare. You'll also be able to join a separate Medicare drug plan.</li></ul>During this period, you can't:<ul><li>Switch from Original Medicare to a Medicare Advantage Plan.</li><li>Join a separate Medicare drug plan if you have Original Medicare.</li><li>Switch from one Medicare drug plan to another if you have Original Medicare.</li></ul>You can only make one change during this period, and any changes you make will be effective the first of the month after the plan gets your request. If you're returning to Original Medicare and joining a separate Medicare drug plan, you don't need to contact your Medicare Advantage Plan to disenroll. The disenrollment will happen automatically when you join the drug plan.</td></tr>
<tr><td>Special Enrollment Period</td><td>Qualifying Life Event</td><td>In most cases, if you join a Medicare Advantage Plan, you must keep it for the calendar year starting the date your coverage begins. However, in certain situations, like if you move or you lose other insurance coverage, you may be able to join, switch, or drop a Medicare Advantage Plan during a Special Enrollment Period.</td></tr>
<tr><td>5-star Special Enrollment Period</td><td>December 8 to November 30 the following year

Note: You can only switch plans once during this period.</td><td>Medicare uses ratings from 1–5 stars to help you compare plans based on quality and performance.

If a Medicare Advantage Plan, Medicare drug plan, or Medicare Cost Plan with a 5-star quality rating is available in your area, you can use the 5-star Special Enrollment Period to switch from your current Medicare plan to a Medicare plan with a 5-star quality rating.

Visit Medicare.gov for more information.</td></tr>
</table>

Important! If you drop your Medicare Supplement Insurance (Medigap) policy to join a Medicare Advantage Plan, you may not get the same policy back. Rules vary by state and your situation. Also, if you don't drop your Medicare Advantage Plan and return to Original Medicare within 12 months of joining, you may be limited in your ability to get a Medigap policy when you return to Original Medicare. See page 78.

Always review the materials your plan sends you (like the "Annual Notice of Change" and "Evidence of Coverage"), and make sure your plan will still meet your needs for the following year. You can also visit Medicare.gov/plan-compare to compare other available options with your current plan.

Does Medicare offer other types of plans or programs to get health coverage?

Yes, some other plans and programs may be offered in your area. Some provide both Hospital (Part A) and Medical (Part B) coverage, while others provide only Part B coverage. Some also provide Medicare drug coverage. They have some (but not all) of the same rules as Medicare Advantage Plans. However, each has special rules and exceptions, so you should contact any plans you're interested in to get more details.

Cost Plans

Cost Plans are a type of Medicare health plan available in certain, limited areas of the country.

- In general, you can join even if you only have Part B.
- If you have Part A and Part B and go to a non-network provider, Original Medicare covers the services. You'll pay the Part A and Part B coinsurance and deductibles.
- You can join any time the Cost Plan is accepting new members.
- You can leave any time and return to Original Medicare.
- You can join a separate Medicare drug plan or you can get Medicare drug coverage (Part D) from the Cost Plan (if offered). You can choose to get a separate Medicare drug plan even if the Cost Plan offers Medicare drug coverage.

Note: You can only add or drop drug coverage at certain times. See pages 80–81.

To see if there are Cost Plans in your area, visit Medicare.gov/plan-compare. You can contact the plan you're interested in for more information. Your State Health Insurance Assistance Program (SHIP) can also help you. See pages 115–118 for the phone number of your local SHIP. A trusted agent or broker may also be able to help.

Program of All-inclusive Care for the Elderly (PACE)

PACE is a Medicare and **Medicaid** program offered in many states that allows people who otherwise need a nursing home-level of care to remain in the community, like a home, apartment, or other appropriate setting. To qualify for PACE, you must meet these conditions:

- You're 55 or older.
- You live in the **service area** of a PACE organization.
- You're certified by your state as needing a nursing home-level of care.
- At the time you join, you're able to live safely in the community with the help of PACE services.

PACE covers all Medicare- and Medicaid-covered care and services, and other services that the PACE team of health care professionals decides are necessary to improve and maintain your health. This includes drugs, as well as any other **medically necessary** care, like doctor or health care provider visits, transportation, home care, hospital visits, and even nursing home stays when necessary.

If you have Medicaid, you won't have to pay a monthly **premium** for the long-term care portion of the PACE benefit. If you have Medicare but not Medicaid, you'll be charged a monthly premium to cover the long-term care portion of the PACE benefit and a premium for Medicare drug coverage (Part D). However, in PACE, there's never a **deductible** or **copayment** for any drug, service, or care approved by the PACE team of health care professionals.

Visit **Medicare.gov/pace** to see if there's a PACE organization that serves your community.

Medicare Innovation Projects

Medicare develops innovative models, **demonstrations**, and pilot projects to test and measure the effect of potential changes in Medicare. These projects help to find new ways to improve health care quality and reduce costs, and sometimes offer you extra benefits and services. Usually, they operate only for a limited time and for a specific group of people and/or are offered only in specific areas. Examples of current models, demonstrations, and pilot projects include innovations in primary care, care related to specific procedures (like hip and knee replacements), cancer care, **skilled nursing facility** or rehabilitation care, and care for people with End-Stage Renal Disease (ESRD). Ask your doctor if they participate in these models, and what it means for your care. To learn more about the current Medicare models, demonstrations, and pilot projects, call 1-800-MEDICARE (1-800-633-4227). TTY users can call 1-877-486-2048.

SECTION 5

Medicare Supplement Insurance (Medigap)

How does Medigap work?

Original Medicare pays for much, but not all, of the cost for covered health care services and supplies. Medicare Supplement Insurance (Medigap) policies sold by private companies can help pay some of the remaining health care costs for covered services and supplies, like copayments, coinsurance, and deductibles.

Some Medigap policies also offer coverage for services that Original Medicare doesn't cover, like medical care when you travel outside the U.S. Generally, Medigap doesn't cover long-term care (like care in a nursing home), vision or dental services, hearing aids, eyeglasses, or private-duty nursing.

Medigap plans are standardized

Medigap must follow federal and state laws designed to protect you, and they must be clearly identified as "Medicare Supplement Insurance." Insurance companies can sell you only a "standardized" plan, identified in most states as plans A - D, F, G, and K - N. All plans offer the same basic benefits, but some offer additional benefits so you can choose which one meets your needs. In Massachusetts, Minnesota, and Wisconsin, Medigap plans are standardized in a different way. If you live in one of these states and want more information, visit

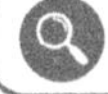 Medicare.gov/medigap-supplemental-insurance-plans.

You can also visit Medicare.gov/publications to view the booklet, "Choosing a Medigap Policy: A Guide to Health Insurance for People with Medicare."

Important! Medigap plans sold to people who are new to Medicare on or after January 1, 2020, aren't allowed to cover the Part B deductible. Because of this, Plans C and F are no longer available to people new to Medicare on or after January 1, 2020. However, if you were eligible for Medicare before January 1, 2020, but not yet enrolled, you may be able to buy Plan C or Plan F. People new to Medicare on or after January 1, 2020, have the right to buy Plans D and G instead of Plans C and F.

Note: See pages 119–122 for definitions of blue words.

How do I compare Medigap plans?

The chart below shows basic information about the different benefits that Medicare Supplement Insurance (Medigap) plans cover for 2023. If a percentage appears, the Medigap plan covers that percentage of the benefit, and you're responsible for the rest.

	Medigap plans									
Benefits	**A**	**B**	**C**	**D**	**F***	**G***	**K**	**L**	**M**	**N**
Medicare Part A coinsurance and hospital costs (up to an additional 365 days after Medicare benefits are used)	100%	100%	100%	100%	100%	100%	100%	100%	100%	100%
Medicare Part B coinsurance or copayment	100%	100%	100%	100%	100%	100%	50%	75%	100%	100%***
Blood (first 3 pints)	100%	100%	100%	100%	100%	100%	50%	75%	100%	100%
Part A hospice care coinsurance or copayment	100%	100%	100%	100%	100%	100%	50%	75%	100%	100%
Skilled nursing facility care coinsurance			100%	100%	100%	100%	50%	75%	100%	100%
Part A deductible		100%	100%	100%	100%	100%	50%	75%	50%	100%
Part B deductible			100%		100%					
Part B excess charges					100%	100%				
Foreign travel emergency (up to plan limits)			80%	80%	80%	80%			80%	80%
							Out-of-pocket limit in 2023**			
							$6,940	$3,470		

*Plans F and G also offer a high-deductible plan in some states. With this option, you must pay for Medicare-covered costs (coinsurance, copayments, and deductibles) up to the deductible amount of $2,700 in 2023 before your policy pays anything. (You can't buy Plans C and F if you were new to Medicare on or after January 1, 2020. See previous page for more information.)

**For Plans K and L, after you meet your out-of-pocket yearly limit and your yearly Part B deductible ($226 in 2023), the Medigap plan pays 100% of covered services for the rest of the calendar year.

***Plan N pays 100% of the Part B coinsurance. You must pay a copayment of up to $20 for some office visits and up to a $50 copayment for emergency room visits that don't result in an inpatient admission.

What else should I know about Medigap?

- Before you can buy Medicare Supplement Insurance (Medigap), you must have Part A and Part B.
- You pay the private insurance company a monthly premium for Medigap in addition to the monthly Part B premium you pay to Medicare. Also, if you buy Medigap and a separate Medicare drug plan from the same company, you may need to make 2 separate premium payments. Contact the company to find out how to pay your premiums.
- A Medigap policy only covers one person. Spouses must buy separate coverage.
- You can't have drug coverage in both Medigap and your Medicare drug plan. See page 89.
- **It's important to compare Medigap policies since the costs can vary between plans offered by different companies for exactly the same coverage, and may go up as you get older. Some states limit Medigap premium costs.**
- In some states, you may be able to buy another type of Medigap policy called Medicare SELECT. Medicare SELECT is a type of Medigap policy sold in some states that requires you to use hospitals and, in some cases, doctors within its network to be eligible for full insurance benefits (except in an emergency). If you buy Medicare SELECT, you have rights to change your mind within 12 months and switch to standard Medigap.

When to buy

- The best time to buy a Medigap policy is during your Medigap Open Enrollment Period. This 6-month period begins the first month you have Medicare Part B (Medical Insurance), **and** you're 65 or older. (Some states have additional Open Enrollment Periods.) **After this enrollment period, you may not be able to buy Medigap. If you're able to buy Medigap, it may cost more.**
- If you delay enrolling in Part B because you have group health coverage based on your (or your spouse's) current employment, your Medigap Open Enrollment Period won't start until you sign up for Part B.
- Federal law generally doesn't require insurance companies to sell Medigap to people under 65. If you're under 65, you might not be able to buy the policy you want, or any policy, until you turn 65. However, some states require Medigap insurance companies to sell Medigap policies to people under 65. If you're able to buy one, it may cost more.

Check with your State Health Insurance Assistance Program (SHIP) (see pages 115–118 for the phone number of your local SHIP), or your State Insurance Department to learn more about your rights to buy a Medigap policy. A trusted agent or broker may also be able to help.

Can I have Medigap and a Medicare Advantage Plan?

- If you're in a Medicare Advantage Plan, it's illegal for anyone to sell you a Medigap policy unless you're switching back to Original Medicare. If you aren't planning to drop your Medicare Advantage Plan, and someone tries to sell you a Medigap policy, report it to your State Insurance Department.
- If you have Medigap and join a Medicare Advantage Plan, you may want to drop Medigap. You can't use Medigap to pay your Medicare Advantage Plan copayments, deductibles, and premiums because Medicare Advantage Plans provide other protections that Medigap doesn't.

Important! **If you want to cancel your Medigap policy, contact your insurance company.** In most cases, if you drop your Medigap policy to join a Medicare Advantage Plan, you may not be able to get the same policy back, or in some cases, any Medigap policy unless you leave your Medicare Advantage Plan during your trial period.

- If you join a Medicare Advantage Plan for the first time, and you aren't happy with the plan, you have a "trial right" under federal law to buy a Medigap policy and a separate Medicare drug plan if you return to Original Medicare within 12 months of joining the Medicare Advantage Plan.

  Note: If you don't drop your Medicare Advantage Plan and return to Original Medicare within 12 months of joining, generally, you must keep your Medicare Advantage Plan for the rest of the year. You can disenroll or change Medicare Advantage Plans during the Open Enrollment Period or if you qualify for a Special Enrollment Period. Depending on the type of Special Enrollment Period, you may or may not have the right to buy a Medigap policy.

  - If you had Medigap before you joined, you may be able to get the same policy back if the company still sells it. If it isn't available, you can buy another policy.
  - If you joined a Medicare Advantage Plan when you were first eligible for Medicare (and you aren't happy with the plan), you can choose from any Medigap policy when you switch to Original Medicare within the first year of joining.
  - Some states provide additional special rights to buy a Medigap policy.

Where can I get more information?

- Call your State Health Insurance Assistance Program (SHIP). See pages 115–118 for the phone number of your local SHIP. A trusted agent or broker in your area may also be able to help.
- Call your State Insurance Department. Call 1-800-MEDICARE (1-800-633-4227) to get the phone number. TTY users can call 1-877-486-2048.
- Visit Medicare.gov/medigap-supplemental-insurance-plans to find policies and pricing in your area.
- Visit Medicare.gov/publications to view the booklet, "Choosing a Medigap Policy: A Guide to Health Insurance for People with Medicare."

SECTION 6

Medicare drug coverage (Part D)

How does Medicare drug coverage work?

Medicare drug coverage (Part D) helps pay for prescription drugs you need. It's optional and offered to everyone with Medicare. Even if you don't take prescription drugs now, consider getting Medicare drug coverage. If you decide not to get it when you're first eligible, and you don't have other creditable prescription drug coverage (like drug coverage from an employer or union) or get Extra Help, **you'll likely pay a late enrollment penalty if you join a plan later.** Generally, you'll pay this penalty for as long as you have Medicare drug coverage (see pages 83-84). To get Medicare drug coverage, you must join a Medicare-approved plan that offers drug coverage. Each plan can vary in cost and specific drugs covered. Visit Medicare.gov/plan-compare to find and compare plans in your area.

There are 2 ways to get Medicare drug coverage (Part D):

1. **Medicare drug plans.** These plans add Medicare drug coverage (Part D) to Original Medicare, some Medicare Cost Plans, some Medicare Advantage Private Fee-for-Service plans, and Medicare Advantage Medical Savings Account plans. You must have Part A and/or Part B to join a separate Medicare drug plan.
2. **Medicare Advantage Plans or other Medicare health plans with drug coverage.** You get your Part A, Part B, and Medicare drug coverage (Part D) through these plans. Remember, you must have Part A and Part B to join a Medicare Advantage Plan, and not all Medicare Advantage Plans offer drug coverage.

In either case, you must live in the service area of the plan you want to join and be lawfully present in the U.S. **Medicare drug plans and Medicare health plans with drug coverage are called "Medicare drug coverage" in this handbook.**

Note: See pages 119–122 for definitions of blue words.

Important! **If you have employer or union coverage**

Call your benefits administrator before you make any changes, or sign up for any other coverage. If you sign up for other coverage, you could lose your employer or union health and drug coverage for you and your dependents. If this happens, you may not be able to get your employer or union coverage back. If you want to know how Medicare drug coverage (Part D) works with other drug coverage you may have, see page 88.

When can I join, switch, or drop a plan?

You can join, switch, or drop a Medicare drug plan or a Medicare Advantage Plan with drug coverage during these times:

- **Initial Enrollment Period.** When you first become eligible for Medicare, you can join a plan. See page 17.
- **Open Enrollment Period.** From October 15 - December 7 each year, you can join, switch, or drop a plan. Your coverage will begin on January 1 (as long as the plan gets your request by December 7).
- **Medicare Advantage Open Enrollment Period.** From January 1 - March 31 each year, if you're in a Medicare Advantage Plan, you can switch to a different Medicare Advantage Plan or switch to Original Medicare (and join a separate Medicare drug plan) once during this time. See page 71.

If you have to pay a premium for Part A and sign up for Part B for the first time during the General Enrollment Period, you can also join a plan from April 1 - June 30. Your coverage will start on July 1.

Special Enrollment Periods

Generally, you must stay in your plan for the entire year. But when certain events happen in your life, like if you move or lose other insurance coverage, you may qualify for a Special Enrollment Period. You may be able make changes to your plan mid-year if you qualify. Check with your plan for more information.

How do I switch plans?

You can switch to a new Medicare drug plan or Medicare Advantage Plan with drug coverage simply by joining another plan during one of the times listed above. Your old drug coverage will end when your new drug coverage begins. You should get a letter from your new plan telling you when your coverage begins, so **you don't need to cancel your old plan.** You can switch plans by calling 1-800-MEDICARE (1-800-633-4227). TTY users can call 1-877-486-2048.

How do I drop my plan?

If you want to drop your separate Medicare drug plan or **Medicare Advantage Plan** with drug coverage and don't want to join a new plan, you can only do so during certain times (see page 80). You can disenroll by calling 1-800-MEDICARE (1-800-633-4227). TTY users can call 1-877-486-2048. You can also send a letter to the plan to tell them you want to disenroll. If you drop your plan and want to join another Medicare drug plan or **Medicare health plan** with drug coverage later, you have to wait for an enrollment period. You may have to pay a late enrollment penalty if you don't have **creditable prescription drug coverage**. See pages 83–84.

Read the information you get from your plan

Review the "Evidence of Coverage" and "Annual Notice of Change" your plan sends you each year. The Evidence of Coverage gives you details about what the plan covers, how much you pay, and more. The Annual Notice of Change includes any changes in coverage, costs, provider networks, **service area**, and more that will be effective in January. If you don't get these important documents in early fall, contact your plan.

How much do I pay?

Your drug costs will vary based on the plan you choose. Remember, plan coverage and costs can change each year. You may have to pay a **premium**, **deductible**, **copayments**, or **coinsurance** throughout the year. Learn more about these costs on the next page.

Your actual drug coverage costs will vary depending on:

- Your prescriptions and whether they're on your plan's list of covered drugs (**formulary**). See page 85.
- What "tier" a drug is in. See page 85.
- Which drug benefit phase you're in (like whether you've met your deductible, or if you're in the catastrophic coverage phase). See page 83.
- Which pharmacy you use (whether it offers preferred or standard cost sharing, is out of network, or is mail order). Your out-of-pocket drug costs may be less at a preferred pharmacy because it has agreed with your plan to charge less.
- Whether you get **Extra Help** paying your Medicare drug costs. See page 91.

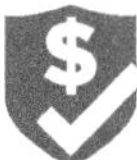

Cost & coverage: Some ways you may be able to lower the cost of your drugs include choosing generics over brand name or paying the non-insurance cost of a drug. Ask your pharmacist—they can tell you if there's a less expensive option available. Check with your doctor to make sure the generic option is best for you.

Monthly premium

Most drug plans charge a monthly fee that varies by plan. You pay this in addition to the Part B **premium**. If you're in a **Medicare Advantage Plan** or a Medicare Cost Plan with drug coverage, the monthly premium may include an amount for drug coverage.

Note: Contact your plan (not Social Security or the Railroad Retirement Board (RRB)) if you want your drug premium deducted from your monthly Social Security or RRB payment. If you want to stop premium deductions and get billed directly, contact your plan.

Important! **If you have a higher income, you might pay more for your Medicare drug coverage.** If your income is above a certain limit (in 2023: $97,000 if you file individually or $194,000 if you're married and file jointly), you'll pay an extra amount in addition to your plan premium (sometimes called "Part D IRMAA"). You'll also have to pay this extra amount if you're in a Medicare Advantage Plan that includes drug coverage. This doesn't affect everyone, so most people won't have to pay an extra amount.

Usually, the extra amount will be deducted from your Social Security or RRB payment. If Medicare or the RRB bills you for the extra amount instead of deducting it from your Social Security or RRB payment, then you must pay the extra amount to Medicare or the RRB, not your plan. If you don't pay the extra amount, you could lose your Medicare drug coverage (Part D). You may not be able to join another plan right away, and you may have to pay a late enrollment penalty for as long as you have drug coverage.

You'll pay Part D IRMAA payments separately, even if your employer or another third party (like a retirement system) pays your plan premiums.

If you have to pay an extra amount and you disagree (for example, you have one or more life-changing events that lower your income), visit **ssa.gov** or call Social Security at 1-800-772-1213. TTY users can call 1-800-325-0778.

Yearly deductible

This is the amount you must pay before your plan begins to pay its share of your covered drugs. Some plans don't have a **deductible**. In some plans that do have a deductible, drugs on some tiers are covered before the deductible.

Copayments or coinsurance

These are the amounts you pay for your covered drugs after the deductible (if the plan has one). You pay your share and your plan pays its share for covered drugs. If you pay **coinsurance**, these amounts may vary because drug plans and manufacturers can change what they charge at any time throughout the year. The amount you pay will also depend on the tier level assigned to your drug. See page 85.

Once you and your plan spend $4,660 combined on drugs (including deductible), you'll generally pay no more than 25% of the cost for prescription drugs until your out-of-pocket spending is $7,400.

Catastrophic coverage

Once your out-of-pocket spending reaches $7,400, you'll automatically get "catastrophic coverage." In most cases, you'll pay no more than 5% of the cost for covered drugs for the rest of the year.

Note: If you get Extra Help, you won't have some of these costs. See pages 91–92.

Important! Visit Medicare.gov/plan-compare to get specific Medicare drug plan and Medicare Advantage Plan costs, and call the plans you're interested in to get more details. For help comparing plan costs, contact your State Health Insurance Assistance Program (SHIP). See pages 115–118 for the phone number of your local SHIP. A trusted agent or broker may also be able to help.

What's the Medicare drug coverage (Part D) late enrollment penalty?

The late enrollment penalty is an amount that's permanently added to your Medicare drug coverage (Part D) premium. You may have to pay a late enrollment penalty if you enroll at any time after your Initial Enrollment Period is over and there's a period of 63 or more days in a row when you don't have Medicare drug coverage or other creditable prescription drug coverage. You'll generally have to pay the penalty for as long as you have Medicare drug coverage.

Note: If you get Extra Help, you don't pay a late enrollment penalty.

There are 3 ways to avoid paying a penalty:

1. **Get Medicare drug coverage (Part D) when you're first eligible for it.** Even if you don't take drugs now, you should consider joining a separate Medicare drug plan or a Medicare Advantage Plan with drug coverage to avoid a penalty. You may be able to find a plan that meets your needs with little to no monthly premiums. See pages 10–14 to learn more about your choices.
2. **Add Medicare drug coverage (Part D) if you lose other creditable coverage.** Creditable prescription drug coverage could include drug coverage from a current or former employer or union, TRICARE, Indian Health Service, the Department of Veterans Affairs, or individual health insurance coverage. Your plan must tell you each year if your non-Medicare drug coverage is creditable coverage. If you go 63 days or more in a row without Medicare drug coverage or other creditable prescription drug coverage, you may have to pay a penalty if you sign up for Medicare drug coverage later.
3. **Keep records showing when you had other creditable drug coverage, and tell your plan when they ask about it.** If you don't tell your plan about your previous creditable prescription drug coverage, you may have to pay a penalty for as long as you have Medicare drug coverage.

How much more will I pay for a late enrollment penalty?
The cost of the late enrollment penalty depends on how long you didn't have creditable prescription drug coverage. Currently, the late enrollment penalty is calculated by multiplying 1% of the "national base beneficiary premium" ($32.74 in 2023) by the number of full, uncovered months that you were eligible but didn't have Medicare drug coverage (Part D) and went without other creditable prescription drug coverage. The final amount is rounded to the nearest $.10 and added to your monthly premium. Since the "national base beneficiary premium" may increase each year, the penalty amount may also increase each year. After you get Medicare drug coverage, the plan will tell you if you owe a penalty and what your premium will be.

Example:
Mrs. Martinez is currently eligible for Medicare, and her Initial Enrollment Period ended on May 31, 2019. She doesn't have prescription drug coverage from any other source. She didn't join by May 31, 2019, and instead joined during the Open Enrollment Period that ended December 7, 2021. Her drug coverage was effective January 1, 2022.

2022
Since Mrs. Martinez was without creditable prescription drug coverage from June 2019–December 2021, her penalty in 2022 was 31% (1% for each of the 31 months) of $33.37 (the national base beneficiary premium for 2022) or $10.34. Since the monthly penalty is always rounded to the nearest $0.10, she paid $10.30 each month in addition to her plan's monthly premium.

Here's the math:
.31 (31% penalty) × **$33.37** (2022 base beneficiary premium) = **$10.34**

$10.34 rounded to the nearest $0.10 = **$10.30**

$10.30 = Mrs. Martinez's monthly late enrollment penalty for 2022

2023
In 2023, Medicare recalculated Mrs. Martinez's penalty using the 2023 base beneficiary premium ($32.74). So, Mrs. Martinez's new monthly penalty in 2023 is 31% of $32.74, or $10.14 each month. Since the monthly penalty is always rounded to the nearest $0.10, she still pays $10.10 each month in addition to her plan's monthly premium.

Here's the math:
.31 (31% penalty) × **$32.74** (2023 base beneficiary premium) = **$10.14**

$10.14 rounded to the nearest $0.10 = **$10.10**

$10.10 = Mrs. Martinez's monthly late enrollment penalty for 2023

What if I don't agree with the late enrollment penalty?
Your Medicare drug plan or Medicare Advantage Plan with drug coverage will send you a letter stating you have to pay a late enrollment penalty. If you disagree with your penalty, you can request a review (generally within 60 days from the date on the letter). Fill out the "reconsideration request form" you get with your letter by the date listed in the letter. You can provide proof that supports your case, like information about previous creditable prescription drug coverage. If you need help, call your plan.

Which drugs are covered?

All plans must cover a wide range of prescription drugs that people with Medicare take, including most drugs in certain "protected classes," like drugs to treat cancer or HIV/AIDS. Information about a plan's list of covered drugs (called a "formulary") isn't included in this handbook because each plan has its own formulary. A plan can make some changes to its drug list during the year if it follows guidelines set by Medicare. Your plan may change its drug list during the year because drug therapies change, new drugs are released, or new medical information becomes available. Your plan coinsurance may increase for a particular brand name drug or generic drug when the manufacturer raises the price. Your copayment or coinsurance may increase when a plan starts to offer a generic form of a brand name drug, but you continue to take the brand name drug.

Your Medicare drug coverage typically places drugs into different levels called "tiers" on their formularies. Drugs in each tier have a different cost. For example, a drug in a lower tier will generally cost you less than a drug in a higher tier. Check with the plan to see if a drug is covered for your health condition. A plan may cover a drug for one condition but not another.

What happens if my drug is in a higher tier?

In some cases, if your drug is in a higher tier and your prescriber (your doctor or other health care provider who's legally allowed to write prescriptions) thinks you need that drug instead of a similar drug in a lower tier, you or your prescriber can ask your plan for an exception to get a lower coinsurance or copayment for the drug in the higher tier. See page 100 for more information on exceptions.

Plans can change their formularies at any time. Your plan may notify you of any formulary changes that affect drugs you're taking.

Note: Medicare drug coverage (Part D) includes drugs, like buprenorphine, to treat opioid use disorders. It also covers drugs, like methadone, when prescribed for pain. However, Medicare Part A covers methadone when used to treat an opioid use disorder as a hospital inpatient, and Part B now covers methadone when you get it through an opioid treatment program.

Contact your plan for its current formulary, or visit the plan's website. You can also visit Medicare.gov/plan-compare or call 1-800-MEDICARE (1-800-633-4227). TTY users can call 1-877-486-2048.

Important! Each month you fill a prescription, your plan sends you an "Explanation of Benefits" notice. Review your notice and check it for mistakes. Contact your plan if you have questions or find mistakes. If you suspect fraud, call the Medicare Drug Integrity Contractor at 1-877-7SAFERX (1-877-772-3379). See page 106.

Plans may have coverage rules for certain drugs

- **Prior authorization:** You and/or your prescriber must contact your plan before you can fill certain prescriptions. Your prescriber may need to show that the drug is medically necessary for the plan to cover it.

  Plans may also use prior authorization when they cover a drug for only certain medical conditions it's approved for, but not others. When this occurs, plans will likely have alternative drugs on their list of covered drugs (formulary) for the other medical conditions the drug is approved to treat.
- **Quantity limits:** Limits on how much medicine you can get at a time.
- **Step therapy:** You may need to try one or more similar, lower-cost drugs before the plan will cover the prescribed drug.
- **Medication safety checks at the pharmacy:** Before the pharmacy fills your prescriptions, your plan and pharmacy perform additional safety checks, like checking for drug interactions and incorrect dosages. These safety checks also include checking for possible unsafe amounts of opioid pain medications, limiting the day's supply of a first prescription for opioids, and use of opioids at the same time as benzodiazepines (commonly used for anxiety and sleep). Opioid pain medicine (like oxycodone and hydrocodone) can help with certain types of pain, but have risks and side effects (like addiction, overdose, and death). These can increase when you take opioids with certain other drugs, like benzodiazepines, anti-seizure medications, gabapentin, muscle relaxers, certain antidepressants, and drugs for sleeping problems. Check with your doctor or pharmacist if you have questions about risks or side effects.
- **Drug Management Programs:** Medicare drug coverage has programs in place to help you use these opioids and benzodiazepines safely. If your opioid use could be unsafe, for example due to getting opioid prescriptions from multiple doctors or pharmacies, or if you had a recent overdose from opioids, your plan will contact the doctors who prescribed them for you to make sure they're medically necessary and you're using them appropriately.

  If your plan decides your use of prescription opioids and benzodiazepines may not be safe, the plan will send you a letter in advance. This letter will tell you if the plan will limit coverage of these drugs for you, or if you'll be required to get the prescriptions for these drugs only from one doctor or pharmacy you select. You and your doctor have the right to appeal these limitations if you disagree with the plan's decision (see page 99). The letter will also tell you how to contact the plan if you have questions or would like to appeal.

  The opioid safety reviews at the pharmacy and Drug Management Programs generally don't apply if you have cancer or sickle cell disease, are getting palliative or end-of-life care, are in hospice, or live in a long-term care facility.

If you or your prescriber believe that your plan should waive one of these coverage rules, you can ask for an exception. See page 100.

Important tips if you're prescribed opioids:

- Opioid medications can be an important part of pain management, but they also can have serious health risks if misused.
- Medicare covers naloxone, a drug that your doctor may prescribe as a safety measure in case you need to rapidly reverse the effects of an opioid overdose. Talk with your doctor about having naloxone at home.
- Talk with your doctor about your dosage and the length of time you'll be taking opioids. You and your doctor may decide later you don't need to take all of your prescription.
- Talk with your doctor about other options that Medicare covers to treat your pain, like non-opioid medications and devices, physical therapy, acupuncture for lower back pain, individual and group psychotherapy, behavioral health integration services, and more.
- Never take more opioids than prescribed. Also, talk with your doctor about any other pain medicines you're taking.
- Safely store and dispose of unused prescription opioids through your community drug take-back program or your pharmacy mail-back program.

For more information on safe and effective pain management and opioid use, visit Medicare.gov/coverage/pain-management or call 1-800-MEDICARE (1-800-633-4227). TTY users can call 1-877-486-2048.

Can I get automatic prescription refills in the mail?

Some people with Medicare get their drugs through an "automatic refill" service that automatically delivers prescription drugs before they run out. To make sure you still need a prescription before they send you a refill, drug plans may offer a voluntary auto-ship program. Contact your plan for more information.

Medication Therapy Management program

Plans with Medicare drug coverage (Part D) must offer Medication Therapy Management services to help members use their opioid prescription drugs safely at no cost to you, if you meet certain requirements or are in a Drug Management Program. If you qualify, you can get these services to help you understand how to manage your medications and take them safely. Medication Therapy Management services usually include a discussion with a pharmacist or health care provider to review your medications. These services may vary by plan.

Contact your plan for specific details and to see if you're eligible for a Medication Therapy Management program. Or, visit Medicare.gov/plan-compare to find and compare health and drug plans.

Part D coverage for insulin

Part D covers injectable insulin used with either a disposable or non-traditional insulin pump. It also covers certain medical supplies used to inject insulin, like syringes, gauze, and alcohol swabs. You **no longer** have to join a plan that's in the Part D Senior Savings Model to get insulin at a lower cost.

New! Plans can't charge you more than $35 for a one-month supply of each Part D-covered insulin you take, and you don't have to pay a deductible for insulin. This applies to everyone who takes insulin, even if you get Extra Help.

Note: Starting July 1, 2023, similar caps on costs will apply for traditional insulin used in insulin pumps (covered under Part B). Visit Medicare.gov/coverage/insulin to learn more.

How do other insurance and programs work with Medicare drug coverage (Part D)?

Medicaid

If you have Medicare and full Medicaid coverage, Medicare covers your prescription drugs. However, Medicaid may still cover some drugs that Medicare doesn't cover.

Note: You automatically qualify for Extra Help if you have Medicare and Medicaid. See page 92.

Employer or union coverage

This is health coverage from your, your spouse's, or other family member's current or former employer or union. If you have drug coverage based on your current or previous employment, your employer or union will notify you each year to let you know if your drug coverage is creditable. **Keep the information you get.** Call your benefits administrator for more information before making any changes to your coverage.

Note: If you get Medicare drug coverage, you, your spouse, or your dependents may lose your employer or union health coverage.

COBRA

This federal law may allow you to temporarily keep employer or union health coverage after the employment ends or after you lose coverage as a dependent of the covered employee. There may be reasons why you should take Part B instead of, or in addition to, COBRA coverage (see page 18). However, if you take COBRA and you're eligible for Medicare, **COBRA may only pay a small portion of your medical costs**, and you may have to pay most of the costs yourself. Contact your COBRA plan and ask what percent they pay. To avoid unexpected medical bills, you may need to sign up for Medicare right away. Talk with your State Health Insurance Assistance Program (SHIP) for free, personalized help with this decision. See pages 115-118 for the phone number of your local SHIP.

Note: If you have COBRA that includes creditable prescription drug coverage, you'll have a Special Enrollment Period to get Medicare drug coverage (Part D) without paying a penalty when the COBRA coverage ends. If you have questions about Medicare and COBRA, call the Benefits Coordination & Recovery Center at 1-855-798-2627. TTY users can call 1-855-797-2627. A trusted agent or broker may also be able to help.

Medicare Supplement Insurance (Medigap) with drug coverage

Medigap policies can no longer be sold with drug coverage, but if you have an older Medigap policy that was sold with drug coverage, you can keep it. You may choose to join a separate Medicare drug plan because most Medigap drug coverage isn't creditable, and you may pay more if you join a drug plan later. See page 83.

You can't have drug coverage in both Medigap and your Medicare drug plan. If you join a separate Medicare drug plan, tell your Medigap insurance company so they can remove the drug coverage and adjust your premiums. Call your Medigap insurance company for more information.

Note: Keep any creditable prescription drug coverage information you get from your plan. You may need it if you decide to join a separate Medicare drug plan later. Don't send creditable coverage letters or certificates to Medicare.

How does other government insurance work with Medicare drug coverage (Part D)?

The types of insurance listed below are all considered creditable prescription drug coverage. In most cases, it's to your advantage to keep this coverage if you have it.

Federal Employee Health Benefits Program (FEHB)

This is health coverage for current and retired federal employees and covered family members. These plans usually include creditable prescription drug coverage, so you don't need to get Medicare drug coverage (Part D). However, if you decide to get Medicare drug coverage, you can keep your FEHB plan, and in most cases, Medicare will pay first. For more information, visit opm.gov/healthcare-insurance/healthcare, or call the Office of Personnel Management at 1-888-767-6738. TTY users can call 1-800-877-8339. If you're an active federal employee, contact your Benefits Officer. Visit apps.opm.gov/abo for a list of Benefits Officers. You can also call your plan if you have questions.

Veterans' benefits

This is health coverage for veterans and people who have served in the U.S. military. You may be able to get drug coverage through the U.S. Department of Veterans Affairs (VA) program. You may join a separate Medicare drug plan, but if you do, you can't use both types of coverage for the same drug at the same time. For more information, visit va.gov or call the VA at 1-800-827-1000. TTY users can call 711.

CHAMPVA (Civilian Health and Medical Program of the Department of Veterans Affairs)

This is a comprehensive health care program in which the Department of Veterans Affairs (VA) shares the cost of covered health care services and supplies with eligible people with Medicare. You may join a separate Medicare drug plan, but if you do, you won't be able to use the Meds by Mail program which can provide your maintenance drugs at no charge (no premiums, deductibles, and copayments). For more information, visit va.gov/communitycare/programs/dependents/champva or call CHAMPVA at 1-800-733-8387.

TRICARE (military health benefits)

This is a health care program for active-duty service members, military retirees, and their families. **Most people with TRICARE who are entitled to Part A must also have Part B to keep their TRICARE drug benefits.** If you have TRICARE, you don't need to join a separate Medicare drug plan. However, if you do, your Medicare drug plan pays first, and TRICARE pays second.

If you join a Medicare Advantage Plan with drug coverage, your Medicare Advantage Plan and TRICARE may coordinate benefits if your Medicare Advantage Plan network pharmacy is also a TRICARE network pharmacy. Otherwise, you can file your own claim to get paid back for your out-of-pocket costs. For more information, visit tricare.mil, or call the TRICARE Pharmacy Program at 1-877-363-1303. TTY users can call 1-877-540-6261.

Indian Health Service (IHS)

The IHS is the primary health care provider to the American Indian/Alaska Native Medicare population. The Indian health care system, consisting of tribal, urban, and federally operated IHS health programs, delivers several clinical and preventive health services through a network of hospitals, clinics, and other entities. Many Indian health facilities participate in the Medicare drug program (Part D). If you get prescription drugs through an Indian health facility, you'll continue to get them at no cost to you, and your coverage won't be interrupted. Joining a Medicare drug plan or Medicare Advantage Plan with drug coverage may help your Indian health facility because the plan pays the Indian health facility for the cost of your prescription drugs. Talk to your local Indian health benefits coordinator who can help you choose a plan that meets your needs and tell you how Medicare works with the Indian health care system.

Note: If you're getting care through an IHS or tribal health facility or program without being charged, you can continue to do so for some or all of your care. Getting Medicare doesn't affect your ability to get services through the IHS and tribal health facilities.

SECTION 7

Get help paying your health & drug costs

Get Extra Help paying your Medicare drug costs

If you have limited income and resources, you may qualify for help to pay for some health care and drug coverage costs.

Extra Help **is a program to help people with limited income and resources pay Medicare drug costs.** You may qualify for Extra Help if your yearly income and resources are below these limits in 2023:

	Yearly income	Other resources
Single person	less than $20,385	less than $15,510
Married person living with a spouse and no other dependents	less than $27,465	less than $30,950

You may qualify even if you have a higher income (like if you still work, live in Alaska or Hawaii, or have dependents living with you). Resources include money in a checking or savings account, stocks, bonds, mutual funds, and Individual Retirement Accounts (IRAs). Resources **don't** include your home, car, household items, burial plot, up to $1,500 for burial expenses (per person), or life insurance policies.

If you qualify for Extra Help and join a separate Medicare drug plan or Medicare Advantage Plan with Medicare drug coverage (Part D):

- You'll get help paying your drug coverage costs.
- You won't pay a late enrollment penalty.

Note: Extra Help isn't available in Puerto Rico, the U.S. Virgin Islands, Guam, the Northern Mariana Islands, or American Samoa. See page 96 for information about programs available in those areas.

Note: See pages 119–122 for definitions of blue words.

Cost & coverage: Most people with Medicare can only make changes to their drug coverage at certain times of the year. If you have Medicaid or get Extra Help, you may be able to make changes to your drug coverage one time during each of these periods:

- January - March
- April - June
- July - September

If you make a change, it will begin the first day of the following month. You can't use this Special Enrollment Period October - December. However, all people with Medicare can make changes to their coverage October 15 - December 7. The changes will begin on January 1.

You automatically qualify for Extra Help if you have Medicare and meet any of these conditions:

- You have full Medicaid coverage.
- You get help from your state Medicaid program paying your Part B premiums (in a Medicare Savings Program). See pages 94–96.
- You get Supplemental Security Income (SSI) benefits.

Medicare will mail you a purple letter to let you know you automatically qualify for Extra Help. Keep this for your records. You don't need to apply for Extra Help if you get this letter.

- If you don't already have Medicare drug coverage (Part D), you must get it to use this Extra Help.
- If you don't have drug coverage, Medicare may enroll you in a separate Medicare drug plan so that you'll be able to use the Extra Help. If Medicare enrolls you in a plan, you'll get a yellow or green letter letting you know when your coverage begins, and you'll have a Special Enrollment Period to change plans if you want to join a different plan than the one Medicare enrolled you in.
- Different plans cover different drugs. Check to see if the plan you're enrolled in covers the drugs you use and if you can go to the pharmacies you want. Visit Medicare.gov/plan-compare or call 1-800-MEDICARE (1-800-633-4227) to compare your plan with other plans in your area. TTY users can call 1-877-486-2048.
- If you have Medicaid and live in certain institutions (like a nursing home) or get home- and community-based services, you pay nothing for your covered drugs.

If you don't want to join a separate Medicare drug plan (for example, because you want only your employer or union coverage), call the plan listed in your letter, or call 1-800-MEDICARE (1-800-633-4227). TTY users can call 1-877-486-2048. Tell them you don't want to be in a Medicare drug plan (you want to "opt out"). If you continue to qualify for Extra Help or if your employer or union coverage is creditable prescription drug coverage, you won't have to pay a penalty if you join later.

Important! If you have employer or union coverage and you get Medicare drug coverage (Part D), you may lose your employer or union coverage (for you and your dependents) even if you qualify for Extra Help. Call your employer's benefits administrator before you get Medicare drug coverage.

Drug costs in 2023 for people who qualify are generally no more than $4.15 for each generic drug and $10.35 for each brand-name drug. Look on the Extra Help letters you get, or contact your plan to find out your exact costs.

If you didn't automatically qualify for Extra Help, you can apply any time:

- Visit secure.ssa.gov/i1020/start to apply online.
- Call Social Security at 1-800-772-1213. TTY users can call 1-800-325-0778.

Note: When you apply for Extra Help, you can also begin the application process for a Medicare Savings Program (MSP). These state programs provide help with other Medicare costs. Social Security will send information to your state to initiate an MSP application, unless you tell them not to on the Extra Help application.

To get answers to your questions about Extra Help and help choosing drug coverage, call your State Health Insurance Assistance Program (SHIP). See pages 115–118 for the phone number of your local SHIP. You can also call 1-800-MEDICARE.

What if I need help paying for my Medicare health care costs?

Medicare Savings Programs

If you have limited income and resources, you may be able to get help from your state to pay your Medicare costs if you meet certain conditions.

There are 4 kinds of Medicare Savings Programs:

1. **Qualified Medicare Beneficiary (QMB) Program:** If you're eligible, the QMB Program helps pay for Part A and/or Part B premiums. In addition, Medicare providers aren't allowed to bill you for services and items Medicare covers, including deductibles, coinsurance, and copayments. If you get a bill for these charges, tell your provider or the debt collector that you're in the QMB Program and can't be charged for Medicare deductibles, coinsurance, and copayments. If you've already made payments on a bill for services and items Medicare covers, you have the right to a refund. If you're in a Medicare Advantage Plan, you should also contact the plan to ask them to stop the charges. In some cases, you may be billed a small copayment through Medicaid, if one applies.

   Note: To make sure your provider knows you're in the QMB Program, show both your Medicare and Medicaid or QMB card each time you get care. If you have Original Medicare, you can also give your provider a copy of your "Medicare Summary Notice" (MSN). Your MSN will show you're in the QMB Program and shouldn't be billed. Log into (or create) your secure Medicare account at Medicare.gov to sign up to get your MSNs electronically.

   If your provider won't stop billing you, call 1-800-MEDICARE (1-800-633-4227). TTY users can call 1-877-486-2048. We can also confirm that you're in the QMB Program.

2. **Specified Low-Income Medicare Beneficiary (SLMB) Program:** Helps pay Part B premiums only.
3. **Qualifying Individual (QI) Program:** Helps pay Part B premiums only. Applications are granted on a first come, first-served basis.
4. **Qualified Disabled and Working Individuals (QDWI) Program:** Helps pay Part A premiums only. You may qualify for this program if you have a disability, you're working, and you lost your Social Security disability benefits and premium-free Part A because you returned to work.

If you sign up for the immunosuppressive drug benefit (see page 53) and have limited income and resources, you may qualify for help paying the costs through a QMB, SLMB, or QI Program. Contact your state to apply. If you qualify for a QMB, SLMB, or QI Program, you automatically qualify to get Extra Help paying for Medicare drug coverage (Part D). See pages 91–93.

Important! The names of these programs and how they work may vary by state. Medicare Savings Programs aren't available in Puerto Rico or the U.S. Virgin Islands.

How do I qualify?
In most cases, to qualify for a Medicare Savings Program, you must have income and resources below a certain limit.

States have different limits and ways of counting your income and resources, so check with your State Medical Assistance (Medicaid) office to see if you qualify.

For more information
Contact your state's Medicaid office or visit Medicaid.gov to get information about Medicare Savings Programs. You can call 1-800-MEDICARE (1-800-633-4227) to get the phone number for your state's Medicaid office. TTY users can call 1-877-486-2048.

Medicaid

Medicaid is a joint federal and state program that helps pay health care costs if you have limited income and (in some cases) resources and meet other requirements. Some people qualify for both Medicare and Medicaid.

What does Medicaid cover?
- If you have Medicare and full Medicaid coverage, most of your health care costs are covered. You can get your Medicare coverage through Original Medicare or a Medicare Advantage Plan.
- If you have Medicare and full Medicaid coverage, Medicare covers your prescription drugs. You automatically qualify for Extra Help paying your Medicare drug costs (see page 91). Medicaid may still cover some drugs that Medicare doesn't cover.
- People with full Medicaid coverage may get coverage for services that Medicare doesn't cover or only partially covers, like nursing home care, personal care, transportation to medical services, home- and community-based services, home-delivered meals, and dental, vision, and hearing services.

How do I qualify?
- Medicaid programs vary from state to state. They may also have different names, like "Medical Assistance" or "Medi-Cal."
- Each state has different income and resource requirements.
- Call your state's Medicaid office for more information and to see if you qualify. Visit Medicare.gov/talk-to-someone or call 1-800-MEDICARE to get the phone number.

Medicare-Medicaid Plans

Medicare is working with some states and health plans to offer demonstration plans for certain people who have both Medicare and Medicaid and make it easier for them to get the services they need. They're called Medicare-Medicaid Plans. These plans include drug coverage and are only in certain states. If you're interested in joining a Medicare-Medicaid Plan, visit Medicare.gov/plan-compare to see if one is available in your area.

State Pharmaceutical Assistance Programs

Many states have State Pharmaceutical Assistance Programs that help certain people pay for prescription drugs based on financial need, age, or medical condition. To find out if there's a State Pharmaceutical Assistance Program in your state and how it works, call your State Health Insurance Assistance Program (SHIP). See pages 115–118 for the phone number of your local SHIP. You can also visit **Medicare.gov/pharmaceutical-assistance-program/#state-programs**.

Pharmaceutical Assistance Programs (also called Patient Assistance Programs)

Many major drug manufacturers offer assistance programs for people with Medicare drug coverage (Part D) who meet certain requirements. Visit **Medicare.gov/pharmaceutical-assistance-program** to learn more about Pharmaceutical Assistance Programs.

Program of All-inclusive Care for the Elderly (PACE)

PACE is a Medicare and **Medicaid** program offered in many states that allows people who need a nursing home-level of care to remain in the community. See page 74.

Supplemental Security Income (SSI) benefits

SSI is a cash benefit Social Security pays to people with limited income and resources who are blind, 65 or older, or have a disability. These benefits aren't the same as Social Security retirement benefits. You may be able to get both SSI and Social Security benefits at the same time if your Social Security benefit is less than the SSI benefit amount, due to a limited work history, a history of low-wage work, or both. If you're eligible for SSI, you automatically qualify for **Extra Help**, and are usually eligible for Medicaid.

You can visit **ssabest.benefits.gov**, and use the "Benefit Eligibility Screening Tool" to find out if you're eligible for SSI or other benefits. Call Social Security at 1-800-772-1213 or contact your local Social Security office for more information. TTY users can call 1-800-325-0778.

Note: People who live in Puerto Rico, the U.S. Virgin Islands, Guam, or American Samoa can't get SSI.

Programs for people who live in the U.S. territories

There are programs in Puerto Rico, the U.S. Virgin Islands, Guam, the Northern Mariana Islands, and American Samoa to help people with limited income and resources pay their Medicare costs. Programs vary in these areas. Call your State Medical Assistance (Medicaid) office to learn more. Visit **Medicare.gov/talk-to-someone** or call 1-800-MEDICARE (1-800-633-4227) to get the phone number. TTY users can call 1-877-486-2048.

SECTION 8

Your Medicare rights & protections

What are my Medicare rights?

All people with Medicare have certain rights and protections. You have the right to:

- Be treated with courtesy, dignity, and respect at all times.
- Be protected from discrimination.
- Have your personal and health information kept private.
- Get information in a way you understand from Medicare, health care providers, and, under certain circumstances, contractors.
- Learn about your treatment choices in clear language you can understand, and participate in treatment decisions.
- Get Medicare information and health care services in a language you understand.
- Get your Medicare information in an accessible format, like braille or large print. See "CMS Accessible Communications" on page 123.

  Note: If you need plan information in a language other than English or in an accessible format, contact your plan.
- Get answers to your Medicare questions.
- Have access to doctors, specialists, and hospitals for **medically necessary** services.
- Get Medicare-covered services in an emergency.
- Get a decision about health care payment, coverage of items and services, or drug coverage. When you or your provider files a claim, you'll get a notice letting you know what will and won't be covered. This notice comes from one of these:
  - Medicare
  - Your **Medicare Advantage Plan** (Part C) or other **Medicare health plan**
  - Your Medicare drug plan

  If you disagree with the decision of your claim, you have the right to file an appeal.
  - Request a review (appeal) of certain decisions about health care payment, coverage of items and services, or drug coverage.
  - Be able to file complaints (sometimes called "grievances"), including complaints about the quality of your care.

Note: See pages 119–122 for definitions of blue words.

- ◦ You can file a complaint if you have concerns about the quality of care and other services you get from a Medicare provider.
- ◦ End-Stage Renal Disease (ESRD) Networks and State Survey Agencies work together to help you with complaints (grievances) about your dialysis or kidney transplant care.

Visit Medicare.gov or call 1-800-MEDICARE (1-800-633-4227) to learn more about filing a complaint. TTY users can call 1-877-486-2048.

What are my rights if my plan stops participating in Medicare?

Medicare health and drug plans can decide not to participate in Medicare for the coming year. In these cases, your coverage under the plan will end after December 31. Your plan will send you a letter explaining your options. If this happens:

- You can choose another plan from October 15–December 7. Your coverage will begin January 1.
- **You also have a special right to join another Medicare plan until the last day in February.**
- You may have the right to buy certain Medigap policies within 63 days after your plan coverage ends.

What's an appeal?

An appeal is the action you can take if you disagree with a coverage or payment decision by Medicare or your Medicare plan. For example, you can appeal if Medicare or your plan denies:

- A request for a health care service, supply, item, or drug you think Medicare should cover.
- A request for payment of a health care service, supply, item, or drug you already got.
- A request to change the amount you must pay for a health care service, supply, item, or drug.

You can also appeal:

- If Medicare or your plan stops providing or paying for all or part of a health care service, supply, item, or drug you think you still need.
- An at-risk determination made under a Drug Management Program that limits access to coverage for frequently abused drugs, like opioids and benzodiazepines. See page 86.

If you decide to file an appeal, you can ask your doctor, supplier, or other health care provider for any information that may help your case. This will make your appeal stronger. Keep a copy of everything related to your appeal, including what you send to Medicare or your plan.

How do I file an appeal?

How you file an appeal depends on the type of Medicare coverage you have.

If you have Original Medicare

- Get the "Medicare Summary Notice" (MSN) that shows the item or service you're appealing. See page 59 for more information about MSNs.
- Circle the item(s) on the MSN you disagree with. Write an explanation of why you disagree with the decision. You can write on the MSN or on a separate piece of paper and attach it to the MSN.
- Include your name, phone number, and Medicare Number on the MSN. Keep a copy for your records.
- Send the MSN, or a copy, to the company that handles bills for Medicare (Medicare Administrative Contractor) listed on the MSN. You can include any information you have about your appeal, like information from your health care provider. Or, you can use CMS Form 20027. To view or print this form, visit CMS.gov/cmsforms/downloads/cms20027.pdf, or call 1-800-MEDICARE (1-800-633-4227) to have a copy mailed to you. TTY users can call 1-877-486-2048.
- You must file your appeal by the date in the MSN. If you missed the deadline for appealing, you may still file an appeal and get a decision if you can show good cause for missing the deadline.
- You'll generally get a decision from the Medicare Administrative Contractor within 60 days after they get your request. If Medicare will cover the item(s) or service(s), it will be listed on your next MSN.
- You may have the right to a fast appeal if you think your Medicare services from a hospital or other facility are ending too soon. See page 100.

If you're in a Medicare Advantage or other Medicare health plan

The timeframe for filing an appeal may be different than Original Medicare. To learn more, look at the materials your plan sends you, call your plan, or visit Medicare.gov/claims-appeals/how-do-i-file-an-appeal.

In some cases, you can file a fast appeal. See materials from your plan and on page 100.

If you have a separate Medicare drug plan

You have the right to do all of these (even before you buy a certain drug):

- Get a written explanation for drug coverage decisions (called a "coverage determination") from your Medicare drug plan. A coverage determination is the first decision your Medicare drug plan (not the pharmacy) makes about your benefits. This can be a decision about if your drug is covered, if you met the plan's requirements to cover the drug, or how much you pay for the drug. You'll also get a coverage determination decision if you ask your plan to make an exception to its rules to cover your drug.
- Ask for an exception if you or your prescriber (your doctor or other health care provider who's legally allowed to write prescriptions) believes you need a drug that isn't on your plan's list of covered drugs (formulary).
- Ask for an exception if you or your prescriber believes that your plan should waive a coverage rule (like prior authorization).

- Ask for an exception if you think you should pay less for a higher tier drug because you or your prescriber believe you can't take any of the lower tier drugs for the same condition.

How do I ask for a coverage determination or exception?

You or your prescriber must contact your plan to ask for a coverage determination or an exception. If your network pharmacy can't fill a prescription, the pharmacist will give you a notice that explains how to contact your Medicare drug plan so you can make your request. If the pharmacist doesn't give you this notice, ask for a copy.

If you're asking for a prescription you haven't gotten yet, you or your prescriber may make a standard request or an expedited (fast) request by phone or in writing. If you're asking to get paid back for prescription drugs you already bought, your plan can require you or your prescriber to make the standard request in writing.

You or your prescriber can call or write your plan for an expedited (fast) request. Your request will be expedited if you haven't gotten the prescription and your plan determines, or your prescriber tells your plan, that your life or health may be at risk by waiting.

Important! If you're requesting an exception, your prescriber must provide a statement explaining the medical reason why your plan should approve the exception.

What are my rights if I think my services are ending too soon?

If you're getting Medicare services from a hospital, **skilled nursing facility**, home health agency, comprehensive outpatient rehabilitation facility, or hospice, and you think your Medicare-covered services are ending too soon (or that you're being discharged too soon), you can ask for a fast appeal (also known as an "immediate appeal" or an "expedited appeal"). Your provider will give you a "Notice of Medicare Non-Coverage" before your services end telling you how to ask for a fast appeal. You should read this notice carefully. If you don't get this notice, ask your provider for it. With a fast appeal, an independent reviewer will decide if your covered services should continue. You can contact your Beneficiary and Family Centered Care-Quality Improvement Organization for help with filing an appeal. See page 113.

A fast appeal only covers the decision to end services. You may need to start a separate appeals process for any items or services you may have gotten after the decision to end services. Visit **Medicare.gov/publications** to view the booklet, "Medicare Appeals."

How can I get help filing an appeal?

You can appoint a representative to help you. Your representative can be a family member, friend, advocate, attorney, financial advisor, doctor, or someone else who will act on your behalf. For more information, visit **Medicare.gov/claims-appeals/file-an-appeal/can-someone-file-an-appeal-for-me**. You can also get help filing an appeal from your State Health Insurance Assistance Program (SHIP). See pages 115–118 for the phone number of your local SHIP.

What's an "Advance Beneficiary Notice of Non-coverage" (ABN)?

If you have Original Medicare, your doctor, other health care provider, or supplier may give you a written notice if they think Medicare won't pay for the items or services you'll get. This notice is called an "Advance Beneficiary Notice of Non-coverage," or ABN. The ABN lists the items or services that your doctor or health care provider expects Medicare will not pay for, along with an estimate of the costs for the items and services and the reasons why Medicare may not pay.

What happens if I get an ABN?

- You'll be asked to choose whether to get the items or services listed on the notice.
- If you choose to get the items or services listed on the notice, you're agreeing to pay if Medicare doesn't.
- You'll be asked to sign the notice to say that you've read and understood it.
- Doctors, other health care providers, and suppliers don't have to (but still may) give you a notice for services that Medicare never covers. See page 55.
- An ABN isn't an official denial of coverage by Medicare. If Medicare denies payment, you can still file an appeal once you get the "Medicare Summary Notice" (MSN) showing the item or service in question. However, you'll have to pay for the items or services if Medicare decides that the items or services aren't covered (and no other insurer is responsible for payment).

Can I get an ABN for other reasons?

- You may get a "Skilled Nursing Facility ABN" when the facility believes Medicare will no longer cover your stay or other items and services.
- You may get an ABN if you're getting an off-the-shelf back or knee brace that's included in the DMEPOS Competitive Bidding Program and the supplier isn't a contract supplier. Visit the "Competitive Bidding Program areas & items" page at Medicare.gov for more information.

What if I didn't get an ABN?

If your provider was required to give you this notice but didn't, in most cases, your provider must give you a refund for what you paid for the item or service.

Where can I get more information about ABNs?

Visit Medicare.gov/basics/your-medicare-rights/your-protections to learn more about the different types of ABNs and what to do if you get one.

Note: If you're in a Medicare Advantage Plan, you have the right to ask the plan in advance if it covers a certain service, drug, or supply. Contact your plan to request and submit a pre-service organization determination. The plan's response will include instructions to file a timely appeal, if you want one. You also may get plan directed care. This is when a plan provider refers you for a service or to a provider outside the network without getting an organization determination in advance. See page 65.

Your right to access your personal health information

By law, you or your legal representative generally have the right to view and/or get copies of your personal health information from health care providers who treat you and bill Medicare for your care. You also generally have a right to get this information from health plans that pay for your care, including Medicare.

These types of personal health information include:

- Claims and billing records
- Information related to your enrollment in health plans, including Medicare
- Medical and case management records
- Other records that doctors or health plans use to make decisions about you

Generally, you can get your information on paper or electronically. If your providers or plans store your information electronically, they generally must give you electronic copies, if you ask for them. You have the right to get your information in a timely manner, but it may take up to 30 days to get a response. If your information is electronic, you also may request to have it sent to a third party of your choosing. A third party may be a:

- Health care provider who treats you
- Family member
- Researcher

You may have to fill out a form to request copies of your information and pay a fee. This fee typically can't be more than the total cost of:

- Labor for copying the information requested
- Supplies for creating the copy
- Postage (if you ask your health care provider to mail you a copy)

In most cases, you won't be charged for viewing, searching, downloading, or sending your information through an electronic portal.

For more information, visit **hhs.gov/hipaa/for-individuals/guidance-materials-for-consumers**.

If you need help getting and using your health records, the Office of the National Coordinator (ONC) in the U.S. Department of Health & Human Services (HHS) created "The Guide to Getting & Using Your Health Records." This guide can help you through the process of getting your health records and show you how to make sure your records are accurate and complete, so you can get the most out of your health care. Visit **healthit.gov/how-to-get-your-health-record** to view the guide.

How does Medicare use my personal information?

Medicare protects the privacy of your health information. The next 2 pages describe how Medicare may use and give out your information, and explain how you can get this information.

Notice of Privacy Practices for Original Medicare

This notice describes how medical information about you may be used and disclosed and how you can get access to this information. Please review it carefully.

The law requires Medicare to protect the privacy of your personal medical information. It also requires us to give you this notice so you know how we may use and share ("disclose") the personal medical information we have about you.

We must provide your information to:

- You, to someone you name ("designate"), or someone who has the legal right to act for you (your personal representative)
- The Secretary of the Department of Health & Human Services, if necessary
- Anyone else that the law requires to have it

We have the right to use and provide your information to pay for your health care and to operate Medicare. For example:

- Medicare Administrative Contractors use your information to pay or deny your claims, collect your **premiums**, share your benefit payment with your other insurer(s), or prepare your "Medicare Summary Notice."
- We may use your information to provide you with customer services, resolve complaints you have, contact you about research studies, and make sure you get quality care.

We may use or share your information under these limited circumstances:

- To state and other federal agencies that have the legal right to get Medicare data (like to make sure Medicare is making proper payments and to help federal/state **Medicaid** programs)
- For public health activities (like reporting disease outbreaks)
- For government health care oversight activities (like investigating fraud and abuse)
- For judicial and administrative proceedings (like responding to a court order)
- For law enforcement purposes (like providing limited information to find a missing person)
- For research studies that meet all privacy law requirements (like research to prevent a disease or disability)
- To avoid a serious and imminent threat to health or safety
- To contact you about new or changed Medicare benefits
- To create a collection of information that no one can trace to you
- To health care providers and their business associates for care coordination and quality improvement purposes, like participation in **Accountable Care Organizations (ACOs)**

We don't sell or use and share your information to tell you about health products or services ("marketing"). We must have your written permission (an "authorization") to use or share your information for any purpose that isn't described in this notice.

You may take back ("revoke") your written permission at any time, unless we've already shared information because you gave us permission.

You have the right to:

- See and get a copy of the information we have about you.
- Have us change your information if you think it's wrong or incomplete, and we agree. If we disagree, you may have a statement of your disagreement added to your information.
- Get a list of people who get your information from us. The listing won't cover information that we gave to you, your personal representative, or law enforcement, or information that we used to pay for your care or for our operations.
- Ask us to communicate with you in a different manner or at a different place (for example, by sending materials to a PO Box instead of your home address).
- Ask us to limit how we use your information and how we give it out to pay claims and run Medicare. We may not be able to agree to your request.
- Get a letter that tells you about the likely risk to the privacy of your information ("breach notification").
- Get a separate paper copy of this notice.
- Speak to a Customer Service Representative about our privacy notice. Call 1-800-MEDICARE (1-800-633-4227). TTY users can call 1-877-486-2048.

If you believe your privacy rights have been violated, you may file a privacy complaint with:

- The Centers for Medicare & Medicaid Services (CMS). Visit **Medicare.gov** or call 1-800-MEDICARE.
- The U.S. Department of Health & Human Services (HHS), Office for Civil Rights (OCR). Visit **hhs.gov/hipaa/filing-a-complaint**.

Filing a complaint won't affect your coverage under Medicare.

The law requires us to follow the terms in this notice. We have the right to change the way we use or share your information. If we make a change, we'll mail you a notice within 60 days of the change.

The Notice of Privacy Practices for Original Medicare became effective September 23, 2013.

How can I protect myself from identity theft?

Identity theft happens when someone uses your personal information without your consent to commit fraud or other crimes. Personal information includes things like your name and your Social Security, Medicare, credit card, or bank account numbers, and your online Medicare account user name and password. Guard your cards and protect your Medicare and Social Security numbers. **Keep this information safe.**

Only give personal information, like your Medicare Number, to doctors, insurance companies (and their licensed agents or brokers), or plans acting on your behalf; or trusted people in the community who work with Medicare like your State Health Insurance Assistance Program (SHIP). Don't share your Medicare Number or other personal information with any unsolicited person who contacts you by phone, email, or in person. Medicare, or your Medicare plan representative, will only call you in limited situations:

- A Medicare plan can call you if you're already a member of the plan. The agent who helped you join can also call you.
- A customer service representative from 1-800-MEDICARE (1-800-633-4227) can call you if you've left a message, or a representative said that someone would call you back. TTY users can call 1-877-486-2048.
- If you filed a report of suspected fraud, you may get a call from someone representing Medicare to follow up on your investigation.

If you suspect identity theft, or feel like you gave your personal information to someone you shouldn't have, call the Federal Trade Commission's ID Theft Hotline at 1-877-438-4338. TTY users can call 1-866-653-4261. You can also visit identitytheft.gov to learn more about identity theft and find helpful resources.

How can I protect myself from fraud and medical identity theft?

Medical identity theft is when someone steals or uses your personal information (like your name, Social Security Number, or Medicare Number) to submit fraudulent claims to Medicare and other health insurance companies without your permission. When you get health care services, record the dates on a calendar and save the receipts and statements you get from providers to check for mistakes. If you think you see an error or a provider bills you for services you didn't get, take these steps to find out what was billed:

- Check your "Medicare Summary Notice" (MSN) if you have Original Medicare to see if the service was billed to Medicare. If you're in a Medicare health plan, check the statements you get from your plan.
- Log into (or create) your secure Medicare account at Medicare.gov to view your Medicare claims if you have Original Medicare. Your claims are generally available online within 24 hours after processing. You can also use Medicare's Blue Button to download your claims information. See page 109. You can also call 1-800-MEDICARE.
- If you know the health care provider or supplier, call and ask for an itemized statement. They should give this to you within 30 days.

If you've contacted the provider and you suspect that Medicare is being charged for a service or supply that you didn't get, or you don't know the provider on the claim, call 1-800-MEDICARE.

You can also call 1-800-MEDICARE (1-800-633-4227) if you believe your Medicare Number has been used fraudulently. TTY users can call 1-877-486-2048.

For more information about Medicare fraud, visit Medicare.gov or contact your local Senior Medicare Patrol Program. Learn more about the Senior Patrol Program and find help in your state by going to smpresource.org or call 1-877-808-2468.

Plans must follow marketing rules

Medicare plans and agents must follow certain rules when marketing their plans and getting your enrollment information. They can't ask you for credit card or banking information over the phone or via email, unless you're already a member of that plan. Plans don't need your personal information to provide a quote. Medicare plans can't sign you up for a plan over the phone unless you call them and ask to sign up, or you've given them permission to contact you.

Important! **Call 1-800-MEDICARE to report any plans or agents that:**

- Ask for your personal information over the phone or email
- Call to enroll you in a plan
- Visit you unexpectedly
- Use false information to mislead you

You can also call the Medicare Drug Integrity Contractor (MEDIC) at 1-877-7SAFERX (1-877-772-3379). The MEDIC fights fraud, waste, and abuse in Medicare Advantage Plans and Medicare drug plans.

Fighting fraud can pay

You may get a reward if you help us fight fraud and meet certain conditions. For more information, visit Medicare.gov or call 1-800-MEDICARE.

Investigating fraud takes time

Every tip counts. Medicare takes all reports of suspected fraud seriously. When you report fraud, you may not hear of an outcome right away. It takes time to investigate your report and build a case, but rest assured that your information is helping us protect Medicare.

Who's the Medicare Beneficiary Ombudsman?

A Medicare Beneficiary Ombudsman helps you and your representatives with questions and complaints, and makes sure Medicare information is available to you. You can also provide feedback to the Ombudsman to help improve your experiences with Medicare. Visit Medicare.gov to learn more.

SECTION 9

Get more information

Get personalized help

1-800-MEDICARE (1-800-633-4227)
TTY users can call 1-877-486-2048
Mail us at PO Box 1270, Lawrence, KS 66044

Get information 24 hours a day, including weekends

- Speak clearly and follow the voice prompts to pick the category that best meets your needs.
- Have your Medicare card in front of you, and be ready to give your Medicare Number.
- When prompted for your Medicare Number, speak the numbers and letters clearly one at a time.
- If you need help in a language other than English or Spanish, or need to request a Medicare publication in an accessible format (like large print or braille), let the customer service representative know.

Important!

If you need someone to be able to call 1-800-MEDICARE on your behalf
You can fill out and mail a "Medicare Authorization to Disclose Personal Health Information" form, so Medicare can give your personal health information to someone other than you. Visit Medicare.gov/basics/forms-publications-mailings to find the form or call 1-800-MEDICARE. You can also submit this form online in your Medicare account. Medicare must process the form before the authorization becomes effective.

If your household got more than one copy of "Medicare & You"

If you want to get only one copy of this handbook in the future, call 1-800-MEDICARE. If you want to stop getting paper copies in the mail, you can request this by logging into (or creating) your Medicare account at Medicare.gov.

If you need a new copy of your Medicare card

If you need to replace your card because it's damaged or lost, visit Medicare.gov to log into (or create) your secure Medicare account to print or order an official copy of your Medicare card. You can also call 1-800-MEDICARE and ask for a replacement card to be sent in the mail.

If you need to replace your card because you think that someone else is using your Medicare Number, call 1-800-MEDICARE.

Note: See pages 119–122 for definitions of blue words.

If you moved, contact Social Security

If you recently moved or plan to move, update your address to continue getting important information from Medicare. Call Social Security at 1-800-772-1213. TTY users can call 1-800-325-0778. If you get Railroad Retirement Board (RRB) benefits, call the RRB at 1-877-772-5772. TTY users can call 1-312-751-4701.

State Health Insurance Assistance Programs (SHIPs)

SHIPs are state programs that get money from the federal government to give local health insurance counseling to people with Medicare at no cost to you. SHIPs aren't connected to any insurance company or health plan. They provide free, personalized counseling to you and your family to help with these and other Medicare questions:

- Your Medicare rights
- Billing problems
- Complaints about your medical care or treatment
- Plan comparison and enrollment
- How Medicare works with other insurance
- Finding help paying for health care costs

See pages 115–118 for the phone number of your local SHIP. Contact a SHIP in your state to get free personalized help with your Medicare questions, or learn how to become a volunteer SHIP counselor.

Find general Medicare information online

Visit Medicare.gov

- Get information about the Medicare health and drug plans in your area, including what they cost and what services they provide.
- Find Medicare-participating doctors or other health care providers and suppliers.
- See what Medicare covers, including **preventive services** (like screenings, shots or vaccines, and yearly "Wellness" visits).
- Get Medicare appeals information and forms.
- Get information about the quality of care provided by plans, nursing homes, hospitals, doctors, home health agencies, dialysis facilities, hospices, **inpatient rehabilitation facilities**, and **long-term care hospitals**.
- Look up helpful websites and phone numbers. You can also visit **Medicare.gov/talk-to-someone** to get answers to your Medicare questions.

You can get this handbook in other languages, like Chinese, Korean, or Vietnamese. Visit **Medicare.gov/about-us/information-in-other-languages**.

Get personal Medicare information online

Create your own Medicare account

Visit Medicare.gov to log into (or create) your secure Medicare account. You can also:

- Add your prescriptions and pharmacies to help you better compare Medicare health and drug plans in your area.
- Sign up to get your yearly "Medicare & You" handbook and claims statements, called "Medicare Summary Notices," electronically.
- View your Original Medicare claims as soon as they're processed.
- Print a copy of your official Medicare card.
- See a list of preventive services you're eligible to get in Original Medicare.
- Learn about your Medicare premiums, and pay them online if you get a bill from Medicare.

Medicare's Blue Button®

Medicare's Blue Button makes it easy for you to download your personal health information (like your Part A, Part B, and Part D claims) to a file on your computer or other device. By getting your information through Blue Button, you can:

- Print or email the information to share with others after you've saved the file.
- Import your saved file into other computer-based personal health management tools.

Remember: Treat your personal and health information the same way you treat other confidential information. Before you share, find out how others will use your information, keep it secure, and protect your privacy.

Visit Medicare.gov and log into (or create) your secure Medicare account to use Blue Button today. You can find step-by-step instructions at Medicare.gov/manage-your-health/share-your-medicare-claims-medicares-blue-button.

Blue Button 2.0®

Medicare has a data service that makes it easy for you to share your Part A, Part B, and Part D claim information with a growing list of authorized apps, services, and research programs. You authorize each app individually and you can return to your secure Medicare account online at Medicare.gov any time to change the way an app uses your information.

Once you use your Medicare account to authorize sharing of your information with an app, you can use that app to view your past and current Medicare claims.

For Medicare Advantage Plans, only Part D information is available through this service. If you're in a Medicare Advantage Plan, check with your plan to see if they offer a similar service to Blue Button 2.0.

Medicare keeps a list of authorized apps. To learn more, visit Medicare.gov/manage-your-health/medicares-blue-button-blue-button-20/blue-button-apps.

Compare the quality of health care providers

Visit Medicare.gov/care-compare to find and compare the quality of care health care providers like nursing homes, hospitals, and doctors give their patients and residents. You can find information about providers and facilities based on your individual needs, and get helpful resources to make more informed decisions about where you get your health care. Talk to your doctor or other health care provider when choosing a provider. You can also ask what they think about the quality of care of other providers.

Compare the quality of Medicare health & drug plans

Visit Medicare.gov/plan-compare to find and compare Medicare health and drug plans, including your current plan, if you've already joined one. You can compare the prices based on the drugs you take now and the pharmacies that you choose to use, including monthly and yearly estimated drug costs. An overall star rating for each plan provides details about its quality and performance for the types of services it offers.

Did you know that you can compare the quality of health care providers and Medicare plan services nationwide? Call your State Health Insurance Assistance Program (SHIP). See pages 115–118 for the phone number of your local SHIP.

Medicare is working to better coordinate your care

Medicare continues to look for ways to better coordinate your care and to make sure that you get the best health care possible.

Here are examples of how your health care providers can better coordinate your care:

Electronic Health Records

Electronic health records are a history of your medical conditions, health care, and treatment that your doctor, other health care provider, medical office staff, or hospital keeps on a computer.

- They can help lower the chances of medical errors, eliminate duplicate tests, and may improve your overall quality of care.
- Your doctor's electronic health records may be able to link to a hospital, lab, pharmacy, other doctors, or immunization information systems (registries), so the people who care for you can have a more complete picture of your health.

Electronic prescribing

This is an electronic way for your prescribers (your doctor or other health care provider who's legally allowed to write prescriptions) to send your prescriptions directly to your pharmacy. Electronic prescribing can save you money and time, and help keep you safe.

Accountable Care Organizations

An Accountable Care Organization (ACO) is a group of doctors, hospitals, and other health care providers that have teamed up to give you coordinated health care.

> Working as part of an ACO helps your doctors and other health care providers understand your health history, and talk to one another about your care and your health care needs. This may save you time, money, and frustration by avoiding repeated tests and appointments. More coordination also helps prevent medical errors and drug interactions, like if one provider isn't aware of what another has prescribed.

Important! An ACO won't limit your choice of health care providers. If your doctor or other provider is part of an ACO, you still have the right to visit any doctor, hospital, or other provider that accepts Medicare at any time.

In addition, if your primary care provider participates in an ACO, you may be able to get expanded benefits. For example, in some ACOs, your provider may offer more telehealth services. This means you may be able to get some services from home using technology, like your phone or a computer, to communicate in real time with your health care provider.

In addition, a doctor or other provider who is part of an ACO may be able to send their patients for **skilled nursing facility care** or rehabilitation services even if they haven't stayed in a hospital for 3 days first, which is usually a requirement in Medicare. For you to qualify for this benefit, your doctor or other provider has to decide that you need skilled nursing facility care and meet certain other eligibility requirements.

If your primary care provider participates in an ACO and you have Original Medicare, you'll get a written notice and see a poster in their office about their ACO participation. There are now hundreds of ACOs across the country. Log into (or create) your secure Medicare account at **Medicare.gov** and choose a primary care provider who will help manage your health care in an ACO.

Securely sharing your health care information with ACOs

One of the most important benefits of an ACO is that your doctors and other providers can communicate and coordinate your care. To help with that, Medicare allows your health care provider's ACO to ask for certain information about your care. Securely sharing your data in this way helps make sure all the people involved in your care have access to your health information when they need it to help you.

If you don't want Medicare to share your health information with your doctors for care coordination, call 1-800-MEDICARE (1-800-633-4227) and let the representative know. TTY users can call 1-877-486-2048. Medicare may still share general information to measure provider quality.

To learn more about ACOs, visit **Medicare.gov/manage-your-health/coordinating-your-care/accountable-care-organizations** or call 1-800-MEDICARE.

Other ways to get Medicare information

Medicare emails

Visit **Medicare.gov** to create your secure Medicare account. Include your email address to get important reminders and information about Medicare.

Publications

Visit **Medicare.gov/publications** to view, print, or download copies of publications on different Medicare topics. You can also call 1-800-MEDICARE. See page 123 for information about getting publications in accessible formats at no cost.

Social media

Stay up to date and connect with other people with Medicare by following us on Facebook (**facebook.com/Medicare**) and Twitter (**twitter.com/MedicareGov**).

Videos

Visit **YouTube.com/cmshhsgov** to see videos covering different health care topics.

Other helpful contacts

Social Security

Visit ssa.gov to apply for and sign up for Original Medicare, and see if you qualify for Extra Help with Medicare drug costs. Also, when you open a personal "my Social Security" account, you can review your Social Security Statement, verify your earnings, change your direct deposit information, request a replacement Medicare card, update your address, and more. Visit ssa.gov/myaccount to open your personal account. You can also call Social Security at 1-800-772-1213. TTY users can call 1-800-325-0778.

Benefits Coordination & Recovery Center

Contact the Benefits Coordination & Recovery Center at 1-855-798-2627 to report changes in your insurance information or to let Medicare know if you have other insurance. TTY users can call 1-855-797-2627.

Beneficiary and Family Centered Care-Quality Improvement Organization

Contact your Beneficiary and Family Centered Care-Quality Improvement Organization (BFCC-QIO) if you think Medicare coverage for your service is ending too soon (like if your hospital says that you must be discharged and you disagree). You may have the right to a fast appeal if you think your Medicare-covered services are ending too soon. You can also contact them to ask questions or report complaints about the quality of care you got for a Medicare-covered service (and if you aren't satisfied with the way your provider has responded to your concern). Call 1-800-MEDICARE (1-800-633-4227) to get the phone number of your BFCC-QIO. TTY users can call 1-877-486-2048.

Department of Defense

Get information about TRICARE For Life (TFL) and the TRICARE Pharmacy Program.

TFL:
1-866-773-0404, TTY: 1-866-773-0405
tricare.mil/tfl
tricare4u.com

TRICARE Pharmacy Program:
1-877-363-1303, TTY: 1-877-540-6261
tricare.mil/pharmacy
militaryrx.express-scripts.com

Department of Veterans Affairs (VA)

Contact the VA if you're a veteran or have served in the U.S. military and you have questions about veteran benefits.

1-800-827-1000, TTY: 711
va.gov
eBenefits.va.gov

Office of Personnel Management

Get information about the Federal Employee Health Benefits Program for current and retired federal employees.

Federal retirees:
1-888-767-6738, TTY: 711
opm.gov/healthcare-insurance/Guide-Me/Retirees-Survivors

Active federal employees:
Contact your Benefits Officer. Visit apps.opm.gov/abo for a list of Benefits Officers.

Railroad Retirement Board (RRB)

If you get benefits from the RRB, call them to change your address or name, check eligibility, sign up for Medicare, replace your Medicare card, or report a death.

1-877-772-5772, TTY: 1-312-751-4701
rrb.gov

State Health Insurance Assistance Programs (SHIPs)

For free, personalized help with questions about appeals, buying other insurance, choosing a health plan, buying a Medigap policy, and Medicare rights and protections.

Alabama

State Health Insurance Assistance Program (SHIP)
1-800-243-5463

Alaska

Medicare Information Office
1-800-478-6065
TTY: 1-800-770-8973

Arizona

Arizona State Health Insurance Assistance Program (SHIP)
1-800-432-4040

Arkansas

Senior Health Insurance Information Program (SHIIP)
1-800-224-6330

California

California Health Insurance Counseling & Advocacy Program (HICAP)
1-800-434-0222

Colorado

State Health Insurance Assistance Program (SHIP)
1-888-696-7213

Connecticut

Connecticut's Program for Health Insurance Assistance, Outreach, Information and Referral, Counseling, Eligibility Screening (CHOICES)
1-800-994-9422

Delaware

Delaware Medicare Assistance Bureau
1-800-336-9500

Florida

Serving Health Insurance Needs of Elders (SHINE)
1-800-963-5337
TTY: 1-800-955-8770

Georgia

Georgia SHIP
1-866-552-4464 (option 4)

Guam

Guam Medicare Assistance Program (GUAM MAP)
1-671-735-7415

Hawaii

Hawaii SHIP
1-888-875-9229
TTY: 1-866-810-4379

Idaho

Senior Health Insurance Benefits Advisors (SHIBA)
1-800-247-4422

Illinois

Senior Health Insurance Program (SHIP)
1-800-252-8966
TTY: 1-888-206-1327

Indiana

State Health Insurance Assistance Program (SHIP)
1-800-452-4800
TTY: 1-866-846-0139

Iowa

Senior Health Insurance Information Program (SHIIP)
1-800-351-4664
TTY: 1-800-735-2942

Kansas

Senior Health Insurance Counseling for Kansas (SHICK)
1-800-860-5260

Kentucky

State Health Insurance Assistance Program (SHIP)
1-877-293-7447

Louisiana

Senior Health Insurance Information Program (SHIIP)
1-800-259-5300

Maine

Maine State Health Insurance Assistance Program (SHIP)
1-800-262-2232

Maryland

State Health Insurance Assistance Program (SHIP)
1-800-243-3425

Massachusetts

Serving Health Insurance Needs of Everyone (SHINE)
1-800-243-4636
TTY: 1-877-610-0241

Michigan

MMAP, Inc.
1-800-803-7174

Minnesota

Minnesota State Health Insurance Assistance Program/ Senior LinkAge Line
1-800-333-2433

Mississippi

MS State Health Insurance Assistance Program (SHIP)
844-822-4622

Missouri

CLAIM
1-800-390-3330

Montana

Montana State Health Insurance Assistance Program (SHIP)
1-800-551-3191

Nebraska

Nebraska SHIP
1-800-234-7119

Nevada

Nevada Medicare Assistance Program (MAP)
1-800-307-4444

New Hampshire

NH SHIP - ServiceLink Resource Center
1-866-634-9412

New Jersey

State Health Insurance Assistance Program (SHIP)
1-800-792-8820

New Mexico

New Mexico ADRC-SHIP
1-800-432-2080

New York

Health Insurance Information Counseling and Assistance Program (HIICAP)
1-800-701-0501

North Carolina

Seniors' Health Insurance Information Program (SHIIP)
1-855-408-1212

North Dakota

State Health Insurance Counseling (SHIC)
1-888-575-6611
TTY: 1-800-366-6888

Ohio

Ohio Senior Health Insurance Information Program (OSHIIP)
1-800-686-1578
TTY: 1-614-644-3745

Oklahoma

Oklahoma Medicare Assistance Program (MAP)
1-800-763-2828

Oregon

Senior Health Insurance Benefits Assistance (SHIBA)
1-800-722-4134

Pennsylvania

Pennsylvania Medicare Education and Decision Insight (PA MEDI)
1-800-783-7067

Puerto Rico

State Health Insurance Assistance Program (SHIP)
1-877-725-4300
TTY: 1-878-919-7291

Rhode Island

Senior Health Insurance Program (SHIP)
1-888-884-8721
TTY: 401-462-0740

South Carolina

(I-CARE) Insurance Counseling Assistance and Referrals for Elders
1-800-868-9095

South Dakota

Senior Health Information & Insurance Education (SHIINE)
1-800-536-8197

Tennessee

TN SHIP
1-877-801-0044
TTY: 1-800-848-0299

Texas

Health Information Counseling and Advocacy Program (HICAP)
1-800-252-9240

Utah

Senior Health Insurance Information Program (SHIP)
1-800-541-7735

Vermont

Vermont State Health Insurance Assistance Program
1-800-642-5119

Virgin Islands

Virgin Islands State Health Insurance Assistance Program (VISHIP)
1-340-772-7368 St. Croix area;
1-340-714-4354 St. Thomas area

Virginia

Virginia Insurance Counseling and Assistance Program (VICAP)
1-800-552-3402

Washington

Statewide Health Insurance Benefits Advisors (SHIBA)
1-800-562-6900
TTY: 1-360-586-0241

Washington D.C.

DC SHIP
202-727-8370

West Virginia

West Virginia State Health Insurance Assistance Program (WV SHIP)
1-877-987-4463

Wisconsin

WI State Health Insurance Assistance Program (SHIP)
1-800-242-1060
TTY: 711

Wyoming

Wyoming State Health Insurance Information Program (WSHIIP)
1-800-856-4398

SECTION 10

Definitions

Accountable Care Organizations (ACOs)

Groups of doctors, hospitals, and other health care professionals working together to give you high-quality, coordinated service and health care.

Assignment

An agreement by your doctor, provider, or supplier to be paid directly by Medicare, to accept the payment amount Medicare approves for the service, and not to bill you for any more than the Medicare deductible and coinsurance.

Benefit period

The way that Original Medicare measures your use of hospital and skilled nursing facility services. A benefit period begins the day you're admitted as an inpatient in a hospital or skilled nursing facility. The benefit period ends when you haven't gotten any inpatient hospital care (or skilled care in a skilled nursing facility) for 60 days in a row. If you go into a hospital or a skilled nursing facility after one benefit period has ended, a new benefit period begins. You must pay the inpatient hospital deductible for each benefit period. There's no limit to the number of benefit periods.

Coinsurance

An amount you may be required to pay as your share of the cost for services after you pay any deductibles. Coinsurance is usually a percentage (for example, 20%).

Copayment

An amount you may be required to pay as your share of the cost for a medical service or supply, like a doctor's visit, hospital outpatient visit, or prescription drug. A copayment is usually a set amount, rather than a percentage. For example, you might pay $10 or $20 for a doctor's visit or prescription drug.

Creditable prescription drug coverage

Prescription drug coverage (for example, from an employer or union) that's expected to pay, on average, at least as much as Medicare's standard prescription drug coverage. People who have this kind of coverage when they become eligible for Medicare can generally keep that coverage without paying a penalty, if they decide to enroll in Medicare prescription drug coverage later.

Critical access hospital

A small facility located in a rural area more than 35 miles (or 15 miles if mountainous terrain or in areas with only secondary roads) from another hospital or critical access hospital. This facility provides 24/7 emergency care, has 25 or fewer inpatient beds, and maintains an average length of stay of 96 hours or less for acute care patients.

Deductible

The amount you must pay for health care or prescriptions before Original Medicare, your Medicare Advantage Plan, your Medicare drug plan, or your other insurance begins to pay.

Demonstrations

Special projects, sometimes called "pilot programs" or "research studies," that test improvements in Medicare coverage, payment, and quality of care. They usually operate only for a limited time, for a specific group of people, and in specific areas.

Extra Help

A Medicare program to help people with limited income and resources pay Medicare prescription drug program costs, like premiums, deductibles, and coinsurance.

Formulary

A list of prescription drugs covered by a prescription drug plan or another insurance plan offering prescription drug benefits. Also called a drug list.

Inpatient rehabilitation facility

A hospital, or part of a hospital, that provides an intensive rehabilitation program to inpatients.

Lifetime reserve days

In Original Medicare, these are additional days that Medicare will pay for when you're in a hospital for more than 90 days. You have a total of 60 reserve days that can be used during your lifetime. For each lifetime reserve day, Medicare pays all covered costs except for a daily coinsurance.

Long-term care hospital

Acute care hospitals that provide treatment for patients who stay, on average, more than 25 days. Most patients are transferred from an intensive or critical care unit. Services provided may include respiratory therapy, head trauma treatment, comprehensive rehabilitation, and pain management.

Medicaid

A joint federal and state program that helps with medical costs for some people with limited income and (in some cases) resources. Medicaid programs vary from state to state, but most health care costs are covered if you qualify for both Medicare and Medicaid.

Medically necessary

Health care services or supplies needed to diagnose or treat an illness, injury, condition, disease, or its symptoms and that meet accepted standards of medicine.

Medicare Advantage Plan (Part C)

A type of Medicare health plan offered by a private company that contracts with Medicare. Medicare Advantage Plans provide all of your Part A and Part B benefits, with a few exclusions, for example, certain aspects of clinical trials which are covered by Original Medicare even though you're still in the plan. Medicare Advantage Plans include:

- Health Maintenance Organizations
- Preferred Provider Organizations
- Private Fee-for-Service Plans
- Special Needs Plans
- Medicare Medical Savings Account Plans

If you're enrolled in a Medicare Advantage Plan:

- Most Medicare services are covered through the plan
- Most Medicare services aren't paid for by Original Medicare
- Most Medicare Advantage Plans offer prescription drug coverage

Medicare-approved amount

In Original Medicare, this is the amount a doctor or supplier that accepts assignment can be paid. It may be less than the actual amount a doctor or supplier charges. Medicare pays part of this amount and you're responsible for the difference.

Medicare health plan

Generally, a plan offered by a private company that contracts with Medicare to provide Part A and Part B benefits to people with Medicare who enroll in the plan. Medicare health plans include all Medicare Advantage Plans, Medicare Cost Plans, and Demonstration/Pilot Programs. Program of All-inclusive Care for the Elderly (PACE) organizations are special types of Medicare health plans. PACE plans can be offered by public or private companies and provide Part D and other benefits in addition to Part A and Part B benefits.

Medicare plan

Any way other than Original Medicare that you can get your Medicare health or drug coverage. This term includes all Medicare health plans and Medicare drug plans.

Medigap

Medicare Supplement Insurance sold by private insurance companies to fill "gaps" in Original Medicare coverage.

Premium
The periodic payment to Medicare, an insurance company, or a health care plan for health or prescription drug coverage.

Preventive services
Health care to prevent illness or detect illness at an early stage, when treatment is likely to work best (for example, preventive services include Pap tests, flu shots, and screening mammograms).

Primary care doctor
The doctor you see first for most health problems. They make sure you get the care you need to keep you healthy. They also may talk with other doctors and health care providers about your care and refer you to them. In many Medicare Advantage Plans, you must see your primary care doctor before you see any other health care provider.

Referral
A written order from your primary care doctor for you to see a specialist or get certain medical services. In many Health Maintenance Organizations (HMOs), you need to get a referral before you can get medical care from anyone except your primary care doctor. If you don't get a referral first, the plan may not pay for the services.

Service area
A geographic area where the plan accepts members. The plan may limit membership based on where people live. For plans that limit which doctors and hospitals you may use, it's also generally the area where you can get routine (non-emergency) services. The plan may disenroll you if you move out of the plan's service area.

Skilled nursing facility (SNF)
A nursing facility with the staff and equipment to give skilled nursing care and, in most cases, skilled rehabilitative services and other related health services.

Skilled nursing facility (SNF) care
Skilled nursing care and therapy services provided on a daily basis in a skilled nursing facility. Examples of skilled nursing facility care include physical therapy or intravenous injections that can only be given by a physical therapist or a registered nurse.

Accessible Communications

Medicare provides free auxiliary aids and services, including information in accessible formats like braille, large print, data or audio files, relay services and TTY communications. If you request information in an accessible format, you won't be disadvantaged by any additional time necessary to provide it. This means you'll get extra time to take any action if there's a delay in fulfilling your request.

To request Medicare or Marketplace information in an accessible format you can:

1. Call us:
   For Medicare: 1-800-MEDICARE (1-800-633-4227)
   TTY: 1-877-486-2048
2. Send us a fax: 1-844-530-3676
3. Send us a letter:

   Centers for Medicare & Medicaid Services
   Offices of Hearings and Inquiries (OHI)
   7500 Security Boulevard, Mail Stop S1-13-25
   Baltimore, MD 21244-1850
   Attn: Customer Accessibility Resource Staff

Your request should include your name, phone number, type of information you need (if known), and the mailing address where we should send the materials. We may contact you for additional information.

Note: If you're enrolled in a Medicare Advantage Plan or Medicare drug plan, contact your plan to request its information in an accessible format. For Medicaid, contact your State Medical Assistance (Medicaid) office.

Nondiscrimination Notice

The Centers for Medicare & Medicaid Services (CMS) doesn't exclude, deny benefits to, or otherwise discriminate against any person on the basis of race, color, national origin, disability, sex, or age in admission to, participation in, or receipt of the services and benefits under any of its programs and activities, whether carried out by CMS directly or through a contractor or any other entity with which CMS arranges to carry out its programs and activities.

You can contact CMS in any of the ways included in this notice if you have any concerns about getting information in a format that you can use.

You may also file a complaint if you think you've been subjected to discrimination in a CMS program or activity, including experiencing issues with getting information in an accessible format from any Medicare Advantage Plan, Medicare drug plan, state or local Medicaid office, or Marketplace Qualified Health Plans. There are 3 ways to file a complaint with the U.S. Department of Health & Human Services, Office for Civil Rights:

1. **Online:**
   hhs.gov/civil-rights/filing-a-complaint/complaint-process/index.html
2. **By phone:**
   Call 1-800-368-1019. TTY users can call 1-800-537-7697.
3. **In writing:** Send information about your complaint to:
   Office for Civil Rights
   U.S. Department of Health & Human Services
   200 Independence Avenue, SW
   Room 509F, HHH Building
   Washington, D.C. 20201

Looking for help in other languages?

If you, or someone you're helping, has questions about Medicare, you have the right to get help and information in your language at no cost. To talk to an interpreter, call 1-800-MEDICARE (1-800-633-4227).

العربية (Arabic) إن كان لديك أو لدى شخص تساعده أسئلة بخصوص Medicare فإن من حقك الحصول على المساعدة و المعلومات بلغتك من دون أي تكلفة. للتحدث مع مترجم إتصل بالرقم 1-800-MEDICARE (1-800-633-4227).

հայերեն (Armenian) Եթե Դուք կամ Ձեր կողմից օգնություն ստացող անձը հարցեր ունի Medicare-ի մասին, ապա Դուք իրավունք ունեք անվճար օգնություն և տեղեկություններ ստանալու Ձեր նախընտրած լեզվով: Թարգմանչի հետ խոսելու համար զանգահարեք 1-800-MEDICARE (1-800-633-4227) հեռախոսահամարով:

中文 (Chinese-Traditional) 如果您，或是您正在協助的個人，有關於聯邦醫療保險的問題，您有權免費以您的母語，獲得幫助和訊息。與翻譯員交談，請致電 1-800-MEDICARE (1-800-633-4227).

فارسی (Farsi) اگر شما، یا شخصی که به او کمک میرسانید سوالی در مورد اعلامیه مختصر مدیکردارید، حق این را دارید که کمک و اطلاعات به زبان خود به طور رایگان دریافت نمایید. برای مکالمه با مترجم با این شماره زیر تماس بگیر ید 1-800-MEDICARE (1-800-633-4227).

Français (French) Si vous, ou quelqu'un que vous êtes en train d'aider, a des questions au sujet de l'assurance-maladie Medicare, vous avez le droit d'obtenir de l'aide et de l'information dans votre langue à aucun coût. Pour parler à un interprète, composez le 1-800-MEDICARE (1-800-633-4227).

Deutsch (German) Falls Sie oder jemand, dem Sie helfen, Fragen zu Medicare haben, haben Sie das Recht, kostenlose Hilfe und Informationen in Ihrer Sprache zu erhalten. Um mit einem Dolmetscher zu sprechen, rufen Sie bitte die Nummer 1-800-MEDICARE (1-800-633-4227) an.

Kreyòl (Haitian Creole) Si oumenm oswa yon moun w ap ede, gen kesyon konsènan Medicare, se dwa w pou jwenn èd ak enfòmasyon nan lang ou pale a, san pou pa peye pou sa. Pou w pale avèk yon entèprèt, rele nan 1-800-MEDICARE (1-800-633-4227).

Italiano (Italian) Se voi, o una persona che state aiutando, vogliate chiarimenti a riguardo del Medicare, avete il diritto di ottenere assistenza e informazioni nella vostra lingua a titolo gratuito. Per parlare con un interprete, chiamate il numero 1-800-MEDICARE (1-800-633-4227).

日本語 (Japanese) Medicare（メディケア）に関するご質問がある場合は、ご希望の言語で情報を取得し、サポートを受ける権利があります（無料）。通訳をご希望の方は、1-800-MEDICARE (1-800-633-4227) までお電話ください。

한국어(Korean) 만약 귀하나 귀하가 돕는 어느 분이 메디케어에 관해서 질문을 가지고 있다면 비용 부담이 없이 필요한 도움과 정보를 귀하의 언어로 얻을 수 있는 권리가 귀하에게 있습니다. 통역사와 말씀을 나누시려면 1-800-MEDICARE(1-800-633-4227)로 전화하십시오.

Polski (Polish) Jeżeli Państwo lub ktoś komu Państwo pomagają macie pytania dotyczące Medicare, mają Państwo prawo do uzyskania bezpłatnej pomocy i informacji w swoim języku. Aby rozmawiać z tłumaczem, prosimy dzwonić pod numer telefonu 1-800-MEDICARE (1-800-633-4227).

Português (Portuguese) Se você (ou alguém que você esteja ajudando) tiver dúvidas sobre a Medicare, você tem o direito de obter ajuda e informações em seu idioma, gratuitamente. Para falar com um intérprete, ligue para 1-800-MEDICARE (1-800-633-4227).

Русский (Russian) Если у вас или лица, которому вы помогаете, возникли вопросы по поводу программы Медикэр (Medicare), вы имеете право на бесплатную помощь и информацию на вашем языке. Чтобы воспользоваться услугами переводчика, позвоните по телефону 1-800-MEDICARE (1-800-633-4227).

Español (Spanish) Si usted, o alguien que está ayudando, tiene preguntas sobre Medicare, usted tiene el derecho a obtener ayuda e información en su idioma sin costo alguno. Para hablar con un intérprete, llame al 1-800-MEDICARE (1-800-633-4227).

Tagalog (Tagalog) Kung ikaw, o ang isang tinutulungan mo, ay may mga katanungan tungkol sa Medicare, ikaw ay may karapatan na makakuha ng tulong at impormasyon sa iyong lenguwahe ng walang gastos. Upang makipag-usap sa isang tagasalin ng wika, tumawag sa 1-800-MEDICARE (1-800-633-4227).

Tiếng Việt (Vietnamese) Nếu quý vị, hay người mà quý vị đang giúp đỡ, có câu hỏi về Medicare, quý vị sẽ có quyền được giúp và có thêm thông tin bằng ngôn ngữ của mình miễn phí. Để nói chuyện qua thông dịch viên, gọi số 1-800-MEDICARE (1-800-633-4227).

“Medicare & You” isn’t a legal document. Official Medicare Program legal guidance is contained in the relevant statutes, regulations, and rulings.

This product was produced at U.S. taxpayer expense.

Printed in the USA
CPSIA information can be obtained
at www.ICGtesting.com
LVHW062245080923
757547LV00011B/532